Aromatherapy for Babies and Children

Also by Shirley Price:

Aromatherapy Workbook
Practical Aromatherapy
Aromatherapy for Health Professionals
Aromatherapy for Common Ailments
Aromatherapy for People with Hearing Difficulties

Another title by Riverhead Publishing which may interest you:

Carrier Oils for Aromatherapy & Massage, by Len Price

Aromatherapy for Babies and Children

Gentle treatments for health and well-being

Penny Price and Shirley Price

Stratford-upon-Avon, Warwickshire, England

AROMATHERAPY FOR BABIES & CHILDREN
Penny Price
Shirley Price

This edition published by Riverhead Publishing,
Stratford–upon–Avon, England 2005
First published in Great Britain by Thorsons 1996

ISBN 1 874353 03 4

Set in Ehrhardt MT 11 on 13
Printed and bound in Oxford, England

Cover design and artwork: Matthew Price
Photographs (except cover): Johnny Lamsdon

To my children: Eleanor, Edward, Toby and Victor – PP

To my grandchildren: Eleanor, Edward, Toby, Victor, Robert, Camilla, Celia and… to parents and children everywhere – SP

Contents

Acknowledgements

To my four children, without whom this book would not have been possible.

Many thanks to my mother and father, Shirley and Len Price, who have taught me almost everything I know about aromatherapy.
PENNY PRICE

To Penny, whose personal experiences form a major part of the book, and whose happy nature allowed me to do all the correlating of our contributions.

To Len, whose fact-checking has been invaluable to both of us – and whose patience after 50 years of marriage and working with me is a delight.
SHIRLEY PRICE

We both thank Johnny Lamsdon for his photographic skills.

Preface

Aromatherapy is suggested in this book as a viable complementary 'medication' for preventative health care for your child and for use with common minor ailments. The authors do not recommend essential oils as a replacement for a doctor's diagnosis and subsequent medication in any instance, although, because essential oils can be used alongside orthodox medicine, they can be used to complement this type of therapy.

Essential oils used as a result of following the information in this book should be used in the exact quantities shown – that is, in a controlled manner. Only the best quality carriers and essential oils will give lasting benefit to your child. (For the sake of simplicity, 'your child' has been referred to as 'he' throughout the text, with the exception of Chapter 6 on Massage, in which 'she' is used in the interests of balance!)

Read on, learn, and most of all, ENJOY using aromatherapy!

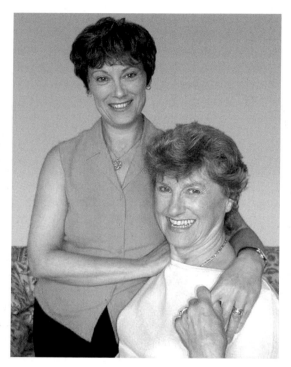

Shirley Price and Penny Price

1

Introduction to Aromatherapy

Aromatherapy is a fairly new word in the English dictionary, having been coined in the 1920s by a French chemist called Gattefossé. It was not in public use until very recently – the last 25 years seeing the word becoming more popular. Because aromatherapy was introduced into Britain by Madame Maury via beauty salons, understanding of the word aromatherapy has been somewhat limited to the general idea of 'massage with a nice smell'! More recently, the general public has seemed content to accept aromatherapy as anything fragranced which may or may not have a remote healing element within it.

Aromatherapy, since its inception, has always been linked with beauty, although most aromatherapists now give a stress-relaxing treatment which has a beneficial action on certain medical conditions. However, the word has lost its original meaning; Gattefossé did not use massage, but used the oils in a more medical way. Nowadays, most people link it only with massage, and many firms have used the name commercially to promote shampoos, bath products and cosmetics which have never even been near a genuine essential oil!

Most aromatherapists have had to face this gross misunderstanding of their very valid profession, and we hope that as Britain enters the next millennium a true clinical awareness of the therapeutic effects of essential oils (as in aromatology) will be much more evident.

A true aromatherapist undergoes a standard of training approved by the aromatherapy associations; unfortunately, as in many other walks of life, there are those who set themselves up to practise or teach after only one or two weekends – mostly spent learning massage rather than the properties of essential oils. Because of this, it is wise to ask the aromatherapist you may wish to visit if he or she is a member of a professional organization.

Shirley and Len Price were the first to introduce a new, advanced form of training called aromatology, in which the student concentrates on theoretical knowledge of the essential oils and *all* the necessary methods of use for professional therapeutic application. This is a great step forward for professional aromatherapists, who come on this course (now taught by the Penny Price Academy of Aromatherapy) to widen both their knowledge and their scope of practice.

Orthodox medicine, although born of natural medicine, relies heavily on synthetic chemicals to effect changes in the body. Most drugs are manufactured to target one particular disease, or one particular organ or part of the body. No one would deny the importance of this type of medicine, which is used on a daily basis to save many lives. However, synthetic molecules in the body do cause side-effects which cannot always be predicted.

There is more to lasting health than identifying illnesses and eradicating them. Health involves the whole body, psychologically as well as physically. Treating one area of a person, much as a mechanic would replace one defunct part of a car engine, does not seem to be the answer when considering the complexity of the quality of life of a human being. As health-conscious individuals, intelligence dictates that a targeted drug cannot always answer our health problems. Surely diet, exercise, rest, fresh air, posture and relaxation must enter the health game as necessary players? Essential oils are very effective within this setting of realistic and holistic health care, stimulating as they do the body's own natural healing mechanisms. A genuine awareness of wholeness is the perfect environment for natural medicine, which can then be active in the best possible way.

We are not suggesting that essential oils be used as an alternative medication (although for minor ailments such as coughs, colds, flu, tonsillitis, etc. they are at the very least equally efficacious compared with orthodox medicine), but when used as complementary care the consumer is offered the best possible health care from every conceivable angle. Essential oils, after accessing the bloodstream, rather than just targeting one portion of the body are carried to every cell in the body, where they are most effective in promoting cellular health, balance and regeneration. Being aware of this approach encourages a holistic outlook on health!

We are products of our 'instant' society, where instant well-being can be achieved with a high-powered drug, conveniently swallowed with no undue thought or effort. In reality, the body is a self-healing mechanism which takes its own time to heal (the immune system can take at least eight weeks to regain strength after a cold virus) and often only needs the gentle stimulation of a natural product (in this case essential oils) and an appropriate lifestyle regime to encourage it back to health. Natural products, when used in a controlled manner, work on the whole body without causing any side-effects on other bodily systems, as orthodox drugs are known to do. If a body is helped naturally in its healing process, then it is much more resilient after the disease has been conquered. If only the disease symptoms themselves are suppressed by drug therapy without involving the body's healing powers, there is a risk of their reappearance a few weeks or months later.

When it comes to our children, we must give serious thought to their quality of life in these times of environmental pollution, fast food, 'convenience' foods and drinks and 'couch potato' attitudes to exercise. Our children are the promise of a brighter future where a healthy diet, exercise and complementary medicine must surely have a place, if only for 'green issue' reasons. Children respond to all the natural elements of life very quickly and should be encouraged to do so in an effort to keep them healthy. Prevention is always better than cure.

As we explore the exciting realm of aromatherapy for children, let your mind be opened to the numerous health opportunities in a sensible way of life.

The Bible and Aromatherapy Today

The history of aromatherapy goes back many, many years. Although it was not in fact called aromatherapy until this century, aromatherapy was (and still is) a part of phytotherapy (therapeutic use of the whole plant). The earliest reference that has been found to plant aromas being used is 18,000 bc, referring to the cave drawings in the caves of Lascaux in the Dordogne[1]. Plant medicine evolved in many eastern countries, though the exact origin of plant medicine is shrouded in the mists of time: history tells us that phytotherapy began in India, Egypt, China and the Middle East all at about the same time, but it is not clear if one part of the world took precedence over the others. We believe that people must have always used plants for eating and for healing. God has put everything we need for our use and our well-being onto this planet; plant medicine is part of this great provision.

Aromatherapy, or 'the smells from plants', has always been used in conjunction with religion. In many religious writings we can read about sweet smells being offered to different gods, being used to appease, to placate, to arouse a god to anger or to promote war against an enemy. In the Bible we can read right from Genesis through to Revelation about aromatic materials being used in all these situations. For example, plant extracts, herbs and spices were mixed together to create anointing oils for priests. All priests and holy men in the Bible were physicians working under the law of God. These priests were responsible for keeping the community happy and healthy, and would look after the spiritual, emotional and physical needs of their people, and we find throughout many religious writings the practice of pouring on oil. Should someone become ill it was the priest's duty to visit and help them become well again, and the priest often used the healing properties of plants and oils, often in conjunction with prayer. (Was it the plants and oils that would restore the person's health, or the person's faith in their particular god or in the priest? Was it the priest's faith in God to answer his prayers and restore health? – who knows!)

In ancient times, the people would tithe to the priest (which meant they would give the priest one-tenth of their income, crops or livestock) and in return the priest would pray for them, guide them in their particular religion and keep them healthy. Should the people become ill it was in the priest's interests to help them become well, because otherwise they would not be able to pay their tithe.

All early physicians were holy men. The sign of surgeons today is a stick with a snake wound around it, which symbolizes the part that Moses had to play when leading the people of Israel through the desert. He was a spiritual and physical leader of his people – with responsibility for *keeping* them healthy. This is very much in contrast to our own system today, where we visit the doctor only when we are sick and the doctor only receives payment from us for the visit and our medication. How much better it is to take care of a healthy body than to look after a sick one!

The priests in olden times, because it was their duty to maintain health among their people, would search out different plants and their therapeutic properties. Thus it is that most of our knowledge about herbal medicine comes from monasteries, where the monks would diligently grow herbs and use them in culinary skills – and also as medicines. It was from such places that Culpeper, the famous 17th-century herbalist, gleaned much of his knowledge.

In Egypt, perfumery was firmly linked to religion. Each deity had his or her own particular fragrance and the statues would be covered with scented oils. The Pharaohs had one perfume for war, one for meditation, one for love, etc. The Egyptians also had extensive knowledge of embalming; the priests forecast that the embalmed bodies would last at least 3,000 years (which they did!). Bandages from such mummies have been known to contain traces of clove, cinnamon and nutmeg. The Greeks took over this knowledge from the Egyptians and catalogued it. This knowledge influenced the Romans. During the Crusades, the Knights Templar and their armies were responsible for taking knowledge of herbal medicine throughout Western Europe, and they brought home with them knowledge that they had gained in the Middle East and the islands of the Mediterranean. In this way much knowledge was spread throughout the world about the marvellous healing properties of plants.

During the bubonic plague, frankincense and pine were burned in the streets. It is well known that frankincense and pine when released into the atmosphere are very antiseptic and disinfectant, and for this reason prevented the spread of the plague to a certain degree. Indoors the people used perfumed candles, pomanders, and garlands containing aromatic oils worn around the neck.

In the Middle Ages many books on the therapeutic uses of plants were written, one being Salmon's *Herbal* (1710). By the late 19th century, many essential oils were in use. At the same time, many healing extracts from plants could be produced synthetically. This was much cheaper and easier than using natural plants – and the use of natural medicines began to decline. Our orthodox medicine springs from the synthetic copies of the original plant medicine.

In the 1920s, Gattefossé, the French chemist who first introduced the term aromatherapy, investigated the antiseptic properties of essential oils because he had discovered the healing properties of lavender. It was not until the late 1950s that essential oils were used in England under the name of aromatherapy, by Marguerite Maury. Beauty therapists were taught by her to use ready-mixed aromatherapy oils in massage. Nowadays we realize that aromatherapy has gone beyond massage only, beyond the use of ready-mixed oils, and beyond the beauty therapy profession – it is presently used in many hospitals in all areas of care, including ante-natal and postnatal care, intensive care, rheumatology, rehabilitation, geriatric care, in the treatment of cancer, HIV and AIDS, and for people with learning disabilities.

The history of aromatherapy is a fascinating subject, as the more one reads about it the more one is convinced of the healing power that is held within plants. Hopefully more and more people will be turning to complementary medicine to use alongside orthodox medicine as we go forward into the 21st century.

What Is an Essential Oil?

Essential oils are natural, liquid mixtures of chemical compounds obtained from aromatic plants; they contain the odorific constituents of the plant. Although given the name 'oils', they are not actually oily to the touch and are completely different from the oils that we normally think of in terms of cooking, such as olive oil, corn oil, etc. Essential oils can be obtained from many different parts of the plants: from the leaves (as in the case of eucalyptus); from twigs or berries (juniper); the bark (cinnamon); wood (sandalwood); roots (ginger); flowers (rose); and from the rinds (lemon) and fruit (black pepper). Different oils can come from different parts of the same plant, for example from the orange tree we can obtain orange oil from the peel, petitgrain oil from the leaf, and neroli oil from the blossom.

These natural extracts are obtained by distillation or by expression. It is important that we understand that the term 'essential oil' applies only to oils gained by one of these two methods, which produce natural and true essential oils – and are safe when used in a controlled manner (*see Chapter 2* for more about these methods of extraction). Other oils can be extracted using solvents, although these, in our opinion, are not safe for use on children or babies.

What Are the Physical Properties of Essential Oils?

Essential oils are volatile – that is, they can evaporate, and do so without leaving a greasy mark on a piece of paper, although some have colour and may stain. This volatility is useful when we want to put drops on our children's pyjamas, for example, to help them to sleep.

Essential oils are divided into three main groups regarding their volatility. Oils in the first group are known as *top notes*; these essential oils evaporate rapidly because they contain a greater percentage of the smallest molecules. They are therefore uplifting, invigorating and energizing when inhaled or introduced to the body via massage or bath. These are the oils we would use as 'pick-me-ups'.

Oils in the second group are known as *middle notes*. Middle notes evaporate a little more slowly than top notes, and because of the balance of smaller and bigger molecules they are more stable and balance the body, keeping all its systems in good working order.

Oils in the third group are called *base notes* and are much the slowest of the three to evaporate because they contain a greater percentage of the heavier molecules. Base notes can help us to relax and de-stress; they are particularly useful when we are trying to help our children to sleep through the night or to calm down. Two or three drops of a base note oil in the bath will achieve wonderful results when it comes to calming your children down (*see page 65*).

The above statements about top, middle and base notes are very general. It is possible, because of the complexity of essential oils, that a base note may contain enough of the smaller, less complicated molecules to have an uplifting effect on the body also. The same can be said for top notes: they may contain a few of the relaxing larger molecules and thus have a sedating effect too, as in bitter orange, which is both uplifting and relaxing. Essential oils, like our own bodies, do not follow any exact rules – they are individuals, like ourselves, and studying them is a lifetime's fascinating occupation!

Essential oils are soluble in vegetable oil, alcohol and various other substances, including the oil which is naturally secreted from our skin. However, they should always be diluted – especially for use on the skin, which is why we dilute them in a bland lotion or a vegetable oil (also known as a carrier) which can then be applied, rubbed or massaged into the skin. Here we have three benefits:

1 the essential oil molecules are very tiny (even the base note ones!) and are absorbed via the hair follicles and pores; they also gain entry in between the skin cells, dissolving in the lipids (natural fatty substances) surrounding the skin cells

2 the lotion or vegetable oil carrier leaves the skin smooth and enriched

3 massage, when used, gives extra healing and soothing benefits.

– a wonderful therapeutic combination.

Cautions

One of the properties of essential oils is that they are inflammable – and this brings us to a note of caution. It is important at all times to ensure that your essential oils are stored with their tops on tightly, in a cool dark place, away from children and animals. They should be kept away from fire or flame of any kind, and in children's bedrooms we would suggest that you do not use a candle burner, but invest in an electric vaporizer available from many good retailers. However, essential oils will not self-combust, so there is no need to be afraid of them if used correctly.

An undiluted essential oil from a reputable supplier should always have a dropper insert in the bottle. This is a very important point to look for when buying an oil – and it helps prevent children from accidentally swallowing any. A pipette type dropper is not safe, as the whole neck of the bottle is accessible when the top is removed.

Therapeutic Qualities of Essential Oils

All essential oils are **antiseptic**, several being more powerful than carbolic acid. In real terms, this means that many essential oils are twice as effective as the average household antiseptic. Some, such as gully gum (*Eucalyptus smithii*), have the added advantage of being analgesic, which means it helps to take pain away. How many times have you wiped your child's knee with a household brand of antiseptic and found that it stings? An essential oil such as rosemary or gully gum has strong antiseptic properties but no stinging side-effect, because they in fact help to dull the pain also. Some essential oils are more antiseptic than others, but every single essential oil that you can buy will have some antiseptic properties. This is useful to know when you are wondering which one to choose in an emergency situation, because you will know that whichever one you do select will have some degree of antiseptic effect. Antiseptic oils can also be useful when one of your children has a cough or a cold. If an oil is put into an electric vaporizer it can help to keep the air sterile and so prevent the spread of airborne infection.

Many oils have **anti-inflammatory** properties. This means that where there is inflammation, pain or swelling the essential oils can be applied in a carrier or in the bath to very good effect. Remember, essential oils balance the body and help to regulate the level of inflammation, so if the tissues are flooded with fluid then the right choice of essential oils can help to normalize the fluid balance within the tissues and, in turn, help to relieve pain. In most cases the essential oils help the body to heal itself – in other words they stimulate the body's own healing mechanisms. Oils that can be used against inflammation include rosemary, tea tree, sweet thyme, chamomile, and lavender. These oils are all very soothing on the skin and the underlying tissues. Someone very wisely said once that the physician's job is to amuse the patient while the body heals itself – this is very true in a great many cases.

Some essential oils are **cicatrizant** – that is, healing on the skin, because they are cell-regenerative. This means that these essential oils help to stimulate the natural reproduction of cell tissue of, for instance, the skin. Excellent oils for helping to accelerate the healing process are geranium, cypress and lavender – and to help reduce any resulting scar tissue, frankincense, myrrh and lavender are good choices. In the case of athlete's foot, as well as treating the actual fungus the essential oils also stimulate the regrowth of healthy human skin, which will take over from the fungus in its own time. This leaves you feeling healthier and also promotes the body's self-healing mechanisms, so that you are less likely to be open to this type of infection a second time.

Some essential oils are **antiviral**, although in fact antiviral is perhaps not quite the right terminology; what these oils do is to stimulate the body's immune system. For instance, it is known that tea tree can help stimulate the production of T-cells in the blood. Many other essential oils produce an immunological response, in other words they produce some slight irritation in the body which helps the body to function normally by strengthening its own immune system. With regular use of essential oils having these properties, the body will be kept in peak form, ready to ward off all types of infections. It is our belief that if you help the body to heal itself and to cope with its own infections instead of letting orthodox medicines do the job for you, then you become healthier and stronger and more able to fight off disease as you meet it. The idea behind inoculation is that when the body receives a little bit of a disease it learns to fight it itself, and therefore when it encounters that same disease in later years the body is able to fight it off. We believe very much that this is what we should be aiming for in this modern world. We need to be strengthening our bodies and using the oils as preventatives, keeping our bodies alert and able to fend for themselves.

Essential oils can also influence the human **hormonal** system. We do not quite know how essential oils manage to do this, but what we do know is that when we inhale essential oils our smell memory is affected, allowing the stress-relieving properties and uplifting properties of the oils to do their work, because the mind is the governor of the body. We also know that when our emotional system is uplifted and de-stressed there is a direct response on the nervous system and the hormonal system, helping them to function on a balanced level and revitalize the body.

Aromatherapists use true natural essential oils because they are the most efficacious. Essences which are natural can achieve results which cannot be gained by the use of synthetic substitutes. The reason for this is that essential oils can be classed as biotic, or pro-life ('for' life). Natural essential oils can be used on living tissue with minimal and sometimes no side-effects, which can be so disastrous in the case of their synthetic alternatives. Also, the human body can accustom itself to the effects of the chemical, synthetic drugs, necessitating ever-increasing dosages. This is not the case with essential oils, which retain their effectiveness even in repeated applications and which can actually strengthen the living tissue while killing off the germs.

Case History

Philip, 14 years old, came to see me [Penny] with tonsillitis. He had been suffering on and off for quite a few years, and each time the doctor prescribed antibiotics. In desperation his mother brought him to us. Having successfully treated another client with the same problem, we decided to use *Eucalyptus smithii*, lemon and tea tree in a throat lotion and in the bath. After four days the boy's mother reported that her son's symptoms had completely disappeared. She was asked to keep using the bath drops as a preventative against further attacks and until he had recovered totally. Two years on, Philip has had no repeat attack, which is apparently very unusual for him and confirms our belief that if we help the body to overcome its own disease using its own resources, then in effect we make it stronger, fitter and better equipped for our environment. By helping the body to heal itself, we are in fact healthier after the illness than we were before it started, because our immune system has been stimulated to deal with other problems which might come our way.

Olfaction and Children

When we sniff, the molecules of the substance being smelled are taken up into our nostrils and dissolve in a sea of mucus at the top of our nasal cavity, where they are picked up by tiny little hairs (or *cilia*). The message that the cilia pick up from the molecules then travels down the olfactory tract and goes into the limbic, or emotional system. The olfactory memory forms part of this limbic system.

As the human olfactory memory is able to store up to 10,000 different smells, it is no wonder that our ancestors were so clever in detecting death or fear just by smelling. Once the message of smell has reached the smell memory and is stored there it can evoke deeply held memories – for instance, the smell of lavender may remind you of your grandmother – which is why a particular scent can 'take you back' many years. Smell can also promote other senses in the body to respond to the message received, for example, when you walk into a supermarket and smell freshly baked bread it can make your salivary glands start producing saliva in readiness for food. Our sense of smell will also protect us from ingesting harmful substances; for instance a glass of milk that has turned sour will be detected by the nose before it ever reaches the lips. Just as the tongue has four receptor sites for different types of tastes, so the olfactory cilia have different receptors for different types of smells. We can experience pepperminty smells and floral smells. We can also experience pungent or putrid smells that are not quite so nice.

Children are born with a wonderful sense of smell. After only a few days a newborn baby will recognize his own mother just by her smell. He has learned to associate food, comfort, warmth and security with one particular smell – that of his own mother. This association can be employed to make a baby get on better with a new babysitter. If the mother wears a certain combination of oils regularly to build up a baby/mother relationship, and then gives the babysitter a tissue sprinkled with those same oils, the baby will accept the babysitter and settle down for her more easily (*see Chapter 5*).

Our ancestors used their sense of smell much more than we do today, because they needed it to find food. They could also smell danger from a long way off and would be able to detect with their sense of smell hostility in a person who was a stranger to them. Their sense of smell always kept them on their guard and was an essential part of their existence … Babies can also detect danger – for instance, some babies will cry in the arms of people with whom they do not feel safe. Nowadays we do not need to detect danger so much because we live in a relatively safe environment.

Today our sense of smell is not used so much – in fact, it is hardly used to its full potential at all. A child still retains this valuable sense of smell, however; children can even detect articles of clothing that belong to their mother, their father or their siblings. Often when trying to calm a young child at night-time, if a parent's garment is put in the cot with the child he will snuggle into the garment and feel the closeness of that particular parent. We can use aromatherapy to help to develop our children's smell receptors, to great benefit.

A child's sense of taste builds up as he gets older; a baby starts with very bland food, then gradually one new food after another is introduced until his taste buds become accustomed to the different tastes he has experienced. We believe this is also true of aromas or smells. When presented with a selection of essential oils, children occasionally reject some of them as being too strong, even though these same aromas are quite enjoyable to an adult. We can conclude from this that some of the stronger aromas are probably not suitable to use on children. From Penny's experience of bringing up her own four children, we have selected 20 essential oils which are ideal for use on children.

Most children love citrus smells, therefore from this class of expressed oils we have chosen lemon, mandarin, orange and bergamot, which are smells children seem to enjoy most. These can be followed by stronger smells such as lavender and chamomile. Smells like sandalwood, cedarwood, frankincense and rose otto are very beautiful, gently aromatic base note oils. Because they do not evaporate so quickly these aromas help children to relax. Oils such as mandarin, rosewood, etc. are referred to by Penny's children as 'happy oils', and are the oils that would generally be used during the day in preference to the base notes, because children need oils which will keep them happy and awake – the relaxing and sedating oils are more useful at bedtime!

As your children grow, other smells can be introduced. As with anything else, our bodies have to be allowed to become accustomed gradually to the different sensations in the world around us. When a baby learns to use his sense of touch, for example, he starts by chewing his own fingers or putting his foot in his mouth; he then experiences reaching out for other objects, and so sensation is built upon sensation and he learns to grow in a steady, progressive way.

Smell Association

We believe that the sense of smell plays a very important role in a child's development. Aromas of our childhood and youth can, in adult life, remind us of things pleasant or unpleasant. Penny has counselled many adults, and by using different types of smells in consultation with them has brought many memories to the surface – some happy, some sad, but all helpful in the healing process.

If we can help our children to learn to associate happy times with happy smells, they can grow up to become more aware of their environment and to be more stable and secure. For instance, Penny used clary sage with lavender each time in the labour ward when having her four children. They remain two of their favourite oils. All four of them relax immediately if these two oils are put in a vaporizer in their rooms. This is very reassuring as, had the births been a terrible experience for any of the children, then they may have associated the smell of clary sage and lavender with unhappiness. However, because they react to these oils in a positive way, Penny believes that they were happy at the time of their birth.

Smell means a lot to human beings. We often base our emotional responses and our judgments on our sense of smell; for example, if we go into a hospital we can sometimes feel sick – even if we are only visiting – and the memory of school cabbage can spoil meals in later life. We can remember, when we smell a 'happy smell', the feeling that that gives us; it can bring back pleasant memories. Circulation is improved, breathing becomes deeper and, by releasing positive hormones and chemicals into the system, we bring therapy to our bodies. This is what we hope to achieve by using essential oils on children, too: we hope they will learn to associate the smells of the essential oils with pleasant experiences like bath time, massage and being close to mum or dad. If parents use essential oils on their children in massage then the mother- or father-child bond will be strengthened. It is good to encourage positive touch with beautiful smells.

Anxiety and Illness

We should mention here the effect which a parent's reaction to illness has upon a growing child. It is right to worry when our children are ill or sick, but sometimes if we over-react, in certain situations, our bodies give off a smell of fear and the child also becomes more frightened about the situation. We need to find a balance between worrying too much and not worrying at all. If we do not worry at all and take no notice when our children fall over, cough or are sick, then they will grow up with the impression that we do not care about them, or that to be ill is not possible and is a bad thing. A quick rub better, a hug and assurance that they are all right (without fussing) is all that is needed in most cases. However, if we over-react to every little situation, the child will grow up playing on every little illness for the attention that he can get. The responsibility of parents is to be loving and kind in all situations and, even when a situation does appear frightening, to try never to give the appearance of being frightened themselves. The child will then be helped to grow up with a balanced attitude towards his own body and his own health, neither over-reacting or under-reacting to a given situation but rather, coping with it in a calm and controlled manner.

A Whole Way of Life

Diet

Children respond amazingly quickly to the natural medicine of essential oils. Possibly the reason for this is that their bodies are innocent and pure – in their short life span to date, they have usually had little opportunity to build up toxic residue from synthetic drugs or a poor or insufficient diet. They have also had minimum pollution exposure to their lungs. Children will continue to respond well if care is taken with their diet, which with children is extremely important, particularly as problems such as eczema and asthma can be deeply exacerbated by the wrong diet. The body is a very fine instrument and will perform wonderfully – if the right balance is maintained. This delicate balancing act is represented in the body's pH level – its acid/alkaline balance. In perfect health the alkaline level is much higher than that of the acid; however, pollutants, stress and a poor diet will tip the balance, making the acid level higher[2]. Too much acidity is detrimental to health, depleting the immune system and leaving the body open to disease. Think of a tooth – an acidic environment attacks the tooth's protective layer, leaving holes for bacteria to get in and multiply – so leading to decay. Foods which tip the balance the wrong way are referred to as acid-forming, so called because once ingested they form acids rather than alkalines in the body, and these acids can cause a great many problems. Acid-forming foods include bread, cakes, biscuits, chocolate, sweets, fizzy pop and (unfortunately!) all the things that children really like.

It is quite difficult to ensure that a child has a decent diet in this day and age. However, it is very important if we are looking at long-term health for our children. When taking their health into account, we need to look not only to essential oils but also to the child's whole lifestyle – diet, exercise, water intake, rest periods and stress. We are what we eat, and as many of today's children seem to be very much plumper than in past generations this can only be due to poor nutrition – over-eating the wrong foods. It seems strange that in an affluent society such as Britain we could be described as having a poor diet when there is so much choice at our disposal. The trouble is that many of the foods families eat today are prepared for convenience and are tinned, frozen or preserved in some way. To encourage your children to eat fresh natural foods in season (with minimum cooking) is obviously the best way to rear a healthy child – with care always being taken to note which foods, if any, produce an adverse reaction. For example, it is known that certain food colourings can exacerbate hyperactivity and that children who are given fresh natural diets soon begin to reduce their hyperactive level to one of normality. We cannot hope to 'cure' our children with aromatherapy or any other type of medicine if we are not prepared to take into account their dietary needs or indeed any other aspect of a healthy lifestyle.

Water

Water is a very important part of a child's diet, as it is an adult's. On the whole, in our western society we drink very little water on its own – it is usually incorporated into squashes, fizzy drinks, tea or coffee. Unfortunately all these forms of taking water into the body are acid-forming. When both our food and fluid intake are acid-forming, the body cells can be irritated. Irritation can lead to inflammation and inflammation can lead to disease or ill health. It is for this reason that we should encourage our children to eat alkaline-forming foods such as fresh fruits and vegetables. As far as water is concerned, although tap water is adequate, bottled or cooled boiled water is best, especially for the very young.

Our bodies are two thirds water and we need water to flush our systems regularly, enabling food to be digested properly – and to help our cells to replace themselves. Because so much of our body is water, our tissues and cells are therefore composed mostly of water. This means we need to drink continually to aid the healthy replacement of cells. Children (and adults) lose water through their skin, more so during hot weather or after exercise when they perspire. We also lose body moisture when we speak and breathe – in fact in one single day we can lose as much as 1 egg-cupful from the sole of each foot! It is therefore common sense that this water needs to be replaced in regular amounts throughout the day in order to replenish the body. Ensuring your child drinks plenty of water, bottled or boiled, will ensure his good health.

Water is also a cleanser, so we need to make sure that our children have an adequate intake. Adequate consumption of water leads to sparkling eyes and clear, healthy skin, and helps the body towards positive growth. It also helps prevent children forming bad habits such as taking fizzy and sweet fruity drinks in excess.

Exercise

As our children grow it is very important that they take sufficient exercise; it is essential for them. As soon as babies are born one of the first things they do is cry, and this is said to exercise or expand the lungs. Kicking and grasping for objects is another way in which babies take exercise. When we take exercise we breathe more deeply into the abdomen and all our cells receive a plentiful supply of oxygen. In other words, the body is well aerated, which helps to build up our cells and tissue growth.

Good posture should always be encouraged in children. Sometimes taller children tend to stoop their shoulders, which in fact can do them physical harm. Children must be encouraged to walk tall and to have good posture when sitting at the table and when bending down to pick up objects. You may have noticed that from a very early age children naturally bend at the knees (rather than at the waist) to pick up objects, but then gradually, unfortunately, they begin to copy their parents and bend from the waist, without bending their knees. Bending at the knees is to be encouraged at all times.

Children have natural boundless energy which encourages their growth and development. It has been said that a top athlete would feel tired after one day of following a toddler around! This makes it easier to understand why parents are exhausted at the end of a day of looking after one (or perhaps more) toddler. If we channel children's energy properly, they will be less hyperactive and less frustrated.

Rest

Just as a child needs a good diet and plenty of exercise, so he needs his rest. An overtired child becomes grumpy and grisly, which in itself can lead to ill health. Therefore plenty of sleep at night and perhaps a nap during the day is very important – especially for pre-school children. If a child's day is planned properly there will be a period for exercise and a period for rest. (A bath in essential oils such as ylang ylang and sandalwood can be very restful and can induce sleep.) Rest is also important for a child's growth and development and good health.

Stress

Stress is another area to consider in a child's life, only this time it must be minimized, not maximized. A stressful child will probably be one who does not take enough exercise, has a poor diet and does not have enough rest. Also, great care should be taken when exposing children to adult conversation. Children are very keen listeners and can often pick up one or two things that an adult is saying – the subject of which may seem harmless for an adult, but be quite worrying for a child; for example, subjects like death, bereavement, loss, child abuse or illness. All these can cause great worry inside a child's mind and can prevent healthy growth, also sleep. A child who overhears a conversation about his grandmother dying may suffer at school and become tearful and pale. It may take many hours of talking through different subjects with him before he finally admits that he is worried about his grandmother dying. This is just one example; we believe that children should be allowed to be children for as long as possible (it is already such a short part of life) and not be subjected to all the stress that a grown up has had to learn to handle.

Smoking

Keeping your child away from a fume-filled environment is essential for healthy cell development and body growth. Many children nowadays suffer from asthma and breathing difficulties, and it is believed that this is partly because they live with adults who smoke. Also our environment is much more polluted nowadays with increased traffic and industry. Obviously if we have the health of our children at heart then we should keep them away from our own pollution in the home so that there is at least one place where they can be totally safe.

Preventative Measures

Use preventative measures whenever possible with your children. This means taking into account everything that we have already discussed in this section – diet, water intake, exercise, rest periods, stress and environmental pollution. These are the fundamentals to health, not only for your child but also for you. Looking after our bodies when they are healthy is much easier than looking after them when they are sick. It therefore seems to make sense to do the best that we can to prevent ourselves and our children from becoming ill. Taking into account all of the above will stand us in very good stead if we want to keep our children as healthy as possible.

1   Ryman D 1984 *The Aromatherapy Handbook*. Daniels, Saffron Walden
2   Bennett G 1992 *Handbook of Clinical Dietetics*. Riverhead, Stratford–upon–Avon

Twenty Essential Oils

Aromatherapy has become quite a confusing issue. Shops, from chemists to department stores, all have their own range of 'aromatherapy' products. Alluring hues of purple, green and peach peep from behind beautifully decorated labels to lure the shopper into purchasing them.

It seems as though 'aromatherapy' means anything that smells nice and looks pretty; and that an 'aromatherapy treatment' is a massage accompanied by a pleasant fragrance!

There is much more to this ancient form of medicine than what is available in the stores suggests, or it would not have survived throughout the centuries. Genuine, true essential oils come from natural plant material via distillation at their source; although they possess their own natural colours, these hues are not visible through the amber glass bottles used for storage and, when diluted 97 per cent for use on the skin, are not noticeable. The supermarket brands (often synthetically based) have vibrant colours added to them to make them more appealing to the public, and have little, if any, of the therapeutic qualities of true essential oils since perfume-quality (inferior) oils are usually used.

True Essential Oils

An essential oil consists only of the volatile molecules of the plant, and these include molecules which are aromatic. The different natural chemicals present in a whole oil each have therapeutic properties which have an effect on the body.

Only a steam-distilled essential oil or an expressed essence can be referred to as a true essential oil in the context of aromatherapy; both these methods of extraction will be discussed later in this chapter. True essential oils are quite difficult to source, so it is always advisable to buy your oils from a qualified and caring aromatherapist or from a company which has a good reputation for the quality of their oils (*see Useful Addresses*).

An oil that is obtained by any other way, such as by the use of solvents or by macerating in an alcohol or a vegetable oil, is not a true essential oil. True essential oils come in small amber glass bottles (7 – 12 ml) with a dropper inside the neck of the bottle and the lids tightly stoppered. Bottles containing a true essential oil should be labelled with the words 'essential oil' and should give the Latin name of the plant from which the oil comes. This indicates that the contents are not mixed with any other product such as a vegetable carrier oil or alcohol. Essential oils which are added to a vegetable oil should not be labelled as essential oils because they are already diluted – and should say so on the label.

Many so-called essential oils, having started their life as pure essential oils, have been adulterated with cheap synthetics to make the essential oil go further. For commercial business reasons many of these oils are man-made, or synthesized in a laboratory. Plant extracts prepared with the use of chemical solvents (used by the perfume industry) usually have the 'prettiest' smells, especially those from blossoms; however, to benefit from the therapeutic qualities of natural essential oils, these should be whole, natural and unadulterated.

Essential oils used for therapeutic purposes come from the parts of many different plants, and from different parts of the same plant, as explained in Chapter 1 (*see page 6*).

Let us look at the two methods by which we can gain true essential oils: distillation and expression.

Distillation

The principle of distillation has been recognized since earliest times (about 3,000 years before Christ). The greatest improvement to the process was made by Avicenna, who about 1,000 years ago lengthened the cooling pipe to enable slower condensation. Since then, slight improvements over the years in techniques and materials have been made – and today it can be quite a sophisticated process. The biggest recent advances in development are the

introduction of the stainless steel still, controllable electric heating of the
water and the steam generator, all of which ensure better control over
the distillation process.

Distillation is an effective method of extracting essential oils from plants.
Sometimes, the plant material has to be crushed or broken up beforehand
in order to make the oil cells more accessible to the steam, as in the case of
sandalwood or fennel seeds. However, plants which carry their essential oil cells
near the surface (such as lavender, melissa), have no need to be broken up first.

To distil the plant material (flowers, leaves, roots, or whatever) it is placed in a
still, resting on a grid (some primitive stills can still be found made from copper
and iron). Steam is directed through the grid and is forced through the tightly
packed plant material, the heat breaking down the essential oil cells and thus
liberating the volatile molecules.

The water vapour (steam) and the plant vapour (essential oil) rise upwards
together, leaving the still and travelling via a pipe into a cooling chamber. As
the two vapours are cooled down inside the pipe they condense and reform
into water and essential oil, which is collected in what is called a florentine vase.
The oil and water usually separate quickly due to the difference in their specific
gravities. Most essential oils are less dense than water and will float to the top –
making separation easy (*see Figure below*). However, a few essential oils (denser
than water) will sink and be tapped off from the bottom of the florentine vase.

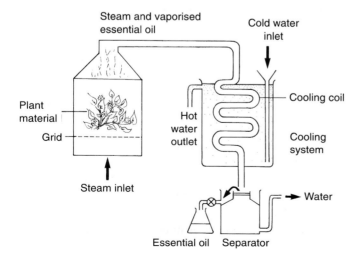

The end result in all cases is what we would term a *true essential oil*. Ideally the plants distilled for therapeutic use are either certificated as being organically grown or have been grown using natural farming methods without pesticides and chemical fertilizers. Wild plants are also used, and these probably give the best quality oil of all.

The distillation time for any particular plant can vary, with lavender being as little as 40 minutes and cedarwood taking several hours. Although the process of distillation sounds very simple, it does require extensive knowledge of both theory and practice, as well as experience. Some plants (with a high yield of oil) are processed in a large still, some (with a low yield of oil) in a small still. The water used for distillation also makes a difference: spring water is best and is used wherever possible. Once used, the water in large stills is usually fed back into the river from which it came, unless it is collected for use as a hydrolat, such as lavender water. For plants containing very little essential oil (e.g. melissa and rose), the water is used over and over again, when it becomes saturated with water-soluble molecules, giving a very concentrated water or hydrolat, which has to be diluted before use.

Expression

Expression is an especially mild process used only for extracting the essential oils from citrus fruits. It is used when steam distillation may damage the end product or because it is cheaper and easier to produce essential oil by this method. Although not distilled, many people refer to these expressed essences as true essential oils.

Expression is simply the pressing of the peel of citrus fruits, which releases the oil. Often the whole, cut fruit is pressed for its juice, and so the oil is not subjected to any heat or any solvent treatment. The colour and other large molecules such as waxes enter into the resultant liquid, which then separates into juice and essential oil.

It is very important that fruits to be expressed for aromatherapy purposes are grown naturally and are not sprayed with chemicals such as pesticides – as these poisonous molecules will end up in the essence.

Other Methods of Extraction

All other methods of plant extraction do not yield what we term essential oils in the aromatherapeutic sense. This is mainly because they involve the addition of solvents during the process. These extracts have names such as absolutes, resinoids and concretes and are not always suitable for use on children's skin (or, in our opinion, on anyone's skin!) as the retained solvent(s) may irritate – depending on the solvent used. They are also thought not to be so beneficial when inhaled, as any solvent present may irritate the lining of the lungs, particularly in an asthmatic. The synthetic perfume material used to fragrance pot-pourri is known to be responsible for the increase in skin and breathing problems today.

All serious aromatherapists would agree that the best oils to use, particularly for children and babies, would be those that have been expressed or steam distilled.

Selected Essential Oils

The following 20 oils have been carefully chosen, based partly on essential oils used in past case studies which have been particularly successful with children. The choice has also been based on the results of a test in which several children were asked to smell certain oils and name their favourites, as for an oil to have a beneficial psychological effect as well as a physiological benefit, the child (just like an adult) needs to enjoy its aroma.

The oils selected have been divided into two main sections: distilled oils and expressed oils (see below). (Those marked with an asterisk [*] are suggested as a result of Penny's personal experience.)

When choosing essential oils for a specific problem it is well to remember that oils are synergistic. This means that when two or three are blended together they work as one oil but produce effects which are greater than that of any one oil used on its own. In effect, in a blend of oils a new material is created, and this will usually give a more effective result.

The effects of the chosen oils have been taken from the well-referenced works, *Alpha to Omega Essential Oils* (Price 1990) and *Aromatherapy for Health Professionals* (Price & Price 1999).

Distilled Essential Oils

Common name	CEDARWOOD
Note	Base
Latin name	*Cedrus atlantica*
Family	Pinaceae (Coniferae)
Description	A tall majestic member of the Coniferae family (which includes both the Pinaceae and Cupressaceae families), this tree bears needles and cones, although it is the wood chippings which are steam distilled, as the wood yields the most oil. There are different types of cedarwood native to different parts of the world. Cedarwood was extracted first in Lebanon and was used by the ancient Egyptians for embalming. The wood was highly prized for building work because the odour repelled insects. It is still used as a temple incense by the Tibetans.
General properties	Cedarwood's antiseptic properties together with its cleansing, refreshing aroma have an excellent effect on respiratory conditions. It is also stimulating to the lymphatic circulation.
Effects and uses	Circulatory: lymph tonic Excretory: cystitis Hair: dandruff, thinning hair (scalp stimulant) Respiratory: bronchitis, coughs and colds Skin: blisters, cradle cap, eczema
Blends aromatically with	bergamot, cypress, marjoram (sweet), rosemary, rosewood
Caution	Not to be used undiluted

Common name	CHAMOMILE (ROMAN)
Note	Middle
Latin name	*Chamaemelum nobile*
Family	Compositae
Description	This small stocky perennial herb, spreading slightly, has a hairy stem, feathery leaves and small daisy-like flowers. Roman chamomile is a member of the Compositae family and is native to the British Isles. The flowers and leaves are steam distilled to give a spicy, apple-like scented oil. There are many varieties of chamomile. Egyptian priests dedicated this herb to the sun; it was also one of the Saxons' nine sacred herbs and was known to be successful in healing the illnesses of nearby plants.
General properties	All chamomiles have a more or less high content of azulene, which is a natural anti-inflammatory agent – German chamomile (*Matricaria recutita*) having the highest. A successful analgesic and nerve sedative, this oil is useful for pain relief. Chamomile is vulnerary (wound-healing) and its digestive qualities have long been appreciated in the form of chamomile tea, used also as a pick-me-up for poorly plants!
Effects and uses	Circulatory: chilblains Digestive: abdominal pain, colic, diarrhoea, indigestion, loss of appetite, travel sickness*, threadworms (itchiness), wind Head: earache, headache, inflamed gums, migraine, teething Nervous: anger, anxiety, crying, depression, distress, hyperactivity, insomnia, irritability, stress Reproductive: hormonal imbalance (teenagers)*, thrush (Candida) Skin: allergies, boils*, burns, chicken pox (inflammation)*, cuts, dermatitis, eczema, inflamed skin, insect bites, nappy rash, psoriasis, scabies, sunburn, wounds
Blends aromatically with	bergamot, lavender, mandarin, marjoram (sweet), ylang ylang
Cautions	None known, although chamomile tea is not recommended for children and people who suffer with allergies. This may be because the tea contains molecules from the whole plant which are not in the essential oil.

Common name	CYPRESS
Note	Middle
Latin name	*Cupressus sempervirens*
Family	Cupressaceae (Coniferae)
Description	An evergreen tree belonging to the Coniferae family, bearing slender branches and having a tall conical shape, native to the eastern Mediterranean. There are many different species of cypress; however *C. sempervirens* has the best therapeutic qualities. The tree bears small flowers and brownish-grey cones, and when not regularly cut for essential oils can reach a height of up to 45 m (150 ft). The wood is hard yet easy to work with, and was used by the Greeks, especially for statues, and by the Phoenicians for ships and houses. The twigs, needles and cones are all steam distilled for this sweet, smokey greenish-yellow oil.
General properties	The most effective property of cypress oil is its action on the vascular system; its styptic qualities are active on circulatory disorders and work as a tonic for the skin and muscular maladies. Its balancing characteristics are soothing to the nerves and cleansing to the mind. Cypress oil is a middle note (*see page 7*) but with sedative qualities.
Effects and uses	Circulatory: chilblains, haemorrhoids, nosebleeds, sluggish circulation, thread veins Digestive: liver tonic Excretory: bedwetting, cystitis Muscular: cramp*, injury (with bleeding) Nervous: crying, hysteria, irritability Respiratory: bronchitis, chest infections, influenza, whooping cough Skin: blisters (astringent), bruises
Blends aromatically with	bergamot, cedarwood, lemon, sandalwood
Cautions	None known

Common name	FRANKINCENSE (OLIBANUM)
Note	Base
Latin name	*Boswellia carteri*
Family	Burseraceae
Description	This small tree, a member of the Burseraceae family, is a native of the Red Sea and has been in use since biblical times. The bark of the tree is cut – to protect itself the tree produces a milky white liquid which hardens to a dark yellow (almost brown) gum. This gum is collected and then steam distilled to give a pale yellow or greenish oil with a fresh sweet balsamic aroma. It has been used in many religions for its calming and clearing effects on the mind, and was once considered to be as precious as gold.
General properties	This oil's antiseptic and regenerative qualities are active on skin conditions, and are especially helpful in reducing scar tissue. Its expectorant qualities aid respiratory conditions. Frankincense is also known as a mind tonic, soothing to the nerves; its aroma imparts a feeling of clarity and quietness useful at times of great stress and anxiety.
Effects and uses	Excretory: kidney tonic* Immune system: stimulant Muscular: aches and pains Nervous: crying, depression, grief, hyperactivity*, stress Respiratory: asthma, bronchitis Skin: burns (helps prevent scarring), chicken pox*, eczema*, nappy rash*, scar tissue, wounds
Blends aromatically with	geranium, ginger, orange (sweet), rose otto, rosewood
Cautions	None known

Common name	GERANIUM
Note	Middle
Latin name	*Pelargonium graveolens*
Family	Geraniaceae
Description	A highly aromatic plant belonging to the Geraniaceae family, there are many varieties of geranium. The aromatic leaves have a lacy edge to them and are slightly hairy. This perennial shrub with pink, unscented flowers can grow up to 1 m (3 ft) tall. The leaves are steam distilled. A potent plant, thought to keep evil spirits away, so often used in window boxes and planters on the doorstep, it is also known to be an insect repellent.
General properties	Uplifting to the spirits, it has deep cleansing properties both to mind and body. It stimulates the lymphatic system and its antiseptic, anti-inflammatory and astringent qualities make it useful for skin conditions. Geranium oil has excellent balancing properties for the whole body and is good for the release of emotions.
Effects and uses	Circulatory: fluid retention, poor, sluggish lymphatic circulation Digestive: diabetes, diarrhoea, gastro-enteritis, jaundice, sluggish liver Hair: dandruff* Head: mouth ulcers*, tonsillitis Muscular: arthritis (analgesic, anti-inflammatory), rheumatism Nervous: agitation, anxiety, crying, depression, hyperactivity, insecurity, neuralgia (analgesic) Skin: acne, allergies*, athlete's foot, blisters, burns, chicken pox*, cold sores, cuts, dermatitis, eczema, impetigo, measles*, nappy rash, ringworm, scars, shingles, ulcers, verrucae*, warts*, wounds
Blends aromatically with	bergamot, frankincense, lavender, lemon, rose otto, rosewood, tea tree
Cautions	None known

Common name	GINGER
Note	Base
Latin name	*Zingiber officinale*
Family	Zingerberaceae
Description	A perennial herb which can grow to 1 m (3 ft) high with a thick, spreading tuberous root, native to eastern Asia. The root is steam distilled after its flowering stem has died off. This plant is now cultivated extensively throughout Nigeria, the West Indies, China and Jamaica (which produces the best ginger for aroma). The sliced or grated root is used frequently in oriental cooking and imparts a spicy/sweet flavour to savoury and sweet dishes. Ginger root has been used for centuries by the Chinese as a herbal remedy for many ailments.
General properties	This spicy aromatic base oil is stimulating to the digestive system; its rubefacient action (increasing local blood circulation) makes it an excellent tonic for muscular circulation in cold weather (in particular for the extremities). Toning and soothing to the digestive system, ginger oil is a powerful anticatarrhal agent useful against chesty winter chills and summer colds and flu.
Effects and uses	Circulatory: poor, sluggish circulation Digestive: abdominal pain, colic, constipation, diarrhoea, flatulence, gastro-enteritis, indigestion, nausea, travel sickness Head: toothache, teething Muscular: aches and pains, cramp*, sprains (analgesic) Nervous: timidity
Blends aromatically with	frankincense, lemon, orange (sweet), rosewood
Cautions	None known

Common name	GULLY GUM EUCALYPTUS
Note	Top
Latin name	*Eucalyptus smithii*
Family	Myrtaceae
Description	There are many different types of eucalyptus tree, all of which are very tall and graceful. When grown for essential oil purposes, however, they are kept well pruned to make them accessible to the people who are picking the leaves, from which the essential oil is obtained. The essential oil cells are deep within the eucalyptus leaf and the leaf has to be crushed before the oil can be accessed.
General properties	Eucalyptus is an effective and versatile antiseptic. *Eucalyptus smithii* is the only eucalyptus which should be used on children, as the popular *Eucalyptus globulus* (blue gum eucalyptus), on sale in many shops, is mostly rectified (that is, altered by chemists to increase the cineole content) and is not suitable for use on children. *E. smithii* is perhaps most commonly used for the relief of chest infections and to facilitate breathing. *E. smithii* is an effective analgesic and is a top note (*see page 7*).
Effects and uses	Circulatory: stimulating locally (i.e., rubefacient) Digestive: threadworms* Excretory: cystitis, kidney infections* Hair: lice*, nits* Muscular: aches and pains, arthritis, injury, spasms* Respiratory: asthma, bronchitis, catarrh, common cold, coughs, croup, hayfever*, sinus trouble Skin: bruises (analgesic), cold sores, high temperature*
Blends aromatically with	lavender, lemon, rosemary
Cautions	None known

Common name	LAVENDER
Note	Middle
Latin name	*Lavandula angustifolia*
Family	Lamiaceae (Labiatae)
Description	A member of the Lamiaceae family, lavender is a small fragrant shrub of square green stems with flowering tops of mostly lilac, although they can also be pink or white. Many an English garden contains a lavender bush somewhere; however, for the essential oil French lavender is the best. This lavender grows above an altitude of 500 m (1,650 ft) on mountainous slopes between the Vercors mountains and the Alps. The lavender is harvested once a year and steam distilled for about 40 minutes. There are many species of lavender, including cross breeds and hybrids which yield more oil but have different therapeutic qualities.
General properties	A very effective balancing middle note, lavender is the most versatile and widely used essential oil. It has been used for centuries as a perfume and to aid sleep. An excellent but gentle antiseptic, analgesic and cell regenerator for wounded tissues, it is very soothing to inflamed skin. Its balancing action is useful for mood swings and moderating hormones – especially in teenagers.
Effects and uses	Circulatory: chilblains, cold feet*, cramp, mottled skin* Digestive: abdominal pain, threadworms (itchiness), thrush (Candida) Head: earache*, headache, teething* Muscular: aches and pains, arthritis, cramp, muscular tension, sports injuries Nervous: anxiety, distress (crying), hyperactivity, insomnia, tantrums Respiratory: bronchial secretions (antiseptic), sore throat*, spasmodic coughing, throat infections Skin: acne, athlete's foot, blisters, bruises (analgesic), burns, chicken pox (anti-inflammatory), cold sores, cradle cap, cuts, eczema, inflammation, insect bites, measles (itchiness), nappy rash, psoriasis, rashes, ringworm, scars, sunburn, wounds

Blends
aromatically with   bergamot, chamomile, eucalyptus, geranium, lemon,
rosemary, rosewood, tea tree, thyme, ylang ylang
Cautions   None known

Common name	MARJORAM (SWEET)
Note	Middle
Latin name	*Origanum majorana*
Family	Lamiaceae
Description	A member of the Lamiaceae family, this small herb grows in sunny places and flowers in the middle of summer. The leaves are grey-green and covered with soft, down-like hair. The essential oil sits in little pockets on the outside of the leaf, protected by the hairs. The oil can be easily washed off by heavy rain, however, so marjoram is best picked when it is dry, as with other members of this family. The aroma of the essential oil varies with climate and the plant is closely related to (and often confused with) oregano. Sweet marjoram is used widely in cooking, especially in Italy.
General properties	Sweet marjoram is an exceptional nerve tonic and its analgesic and anti-inflammatory properties make it invaluable for muscular aches, pains and bruises. Its spicy, camphoraceous odour proves good for chest conditions and head colds. Sweet marjoram is a balancing oil and a good tonic to the digestive system, especially for 'nervous tummies'.
Effects and uses	Circulatory: poor, sluggish circulation Digestive: abdominal pain, colic, diarrhoea, flatulence, gastro-enteritis, indigestion Excretory: bedwetting* Hair: lice* Head: headaches, toothache Muscular: aches and pains, arthritis, cramp, spasm Nervous: agitation, anxiety, day-dreaming, hyperactivity, insomnia, vertigo Respiratory: breathing difficulties, coughs, croup, bronchial infections, sinus troubles, whooping cough
Blends aromatically with	bergamot, cedarwood, chamomile (Roman), tea tree
Cautions	None known

Common name	ROSEMARY
Note	Middle
Latin name	*Rosmarinus officinalis*
Family	Lamiaceae
Description	A strongly aromatic herb which grows up to 1.5 m (5 ft) high with green needle-shaped leaves and pretty pinky/blue flowers. Familiar to the Mediterranean area and popular with the ancient Greeks and Romans to ward off evil spirits and bring peace to the dead. The flowering tops are steam distilled to give an oil with a pungent, sweet herbaceous aroma. Shakespeare termed this plant a 'mind tonic', and ever since his death the churchyard where he is buried is continually fragranced with sprigs of rosemary.
General properties	A multi-talented essential oil, rosemary is analgesic and antispasmodic – very beneficial on tired, aching muscles. A good digestive and a diuretic, poor or slow circulation can be aided by this oil's rubefacient and stimulating actions. A wonderful tonic to the sinuses, rosemary oil sharpens and enlivens sluggish minds.
Effects and uses	Circulatory: stimulating Digestive: colic, constipation, flatulence, indigestion, liver tonic, viral hepatitis Hair: cradle cap, dandruff, dull, thinning hair, lice, nits Head: headaches Muscular: aches and pains, arthritis, cramp, inflammation Nervous: bedwetting, neuralgia, sluggishness (invigorating, stimulates when one is tired or frazzled) Respiratory: bronchitis, common cold, cough, influenza, sinus troubles Skin: bruises, burns, cuts, wounds
Blends aromatically with	cedarwood, eucalyptus, lavender, sandalwood, thyme (sweet)
Cautions	Not to be used undiluted

Common name	ROSE OTTO
Note	Base
Latin name	*Rosa damascena, Rosa centifolia*
Family	Roseacae
Description	The main source of *Rosa centifolia* is Morocco, where it is termed 'the hundred-petalled rose' and is a complex hybrid. *Rosa damascena* is grown mostly in Bulgaria. Only petals are steam distilled and it takes 40 – 50 roseheads to make 1 drop of essential oil. The flowers appear once a year and the harvest period is a mere 40 days, which is another reason why it is so expensive. Rose oil has been regarded for hundreds of years as holy – in the city of Mecca the walls are washed with 500 litres of rose water every year. It is a principal component in leading brands of perfumes and is used extensively in confectionery (for example, in high-quality Turkish Delight).
General properties	Rose oil is a powerful antiseptic, effective on inflammation and respiratory infections, and its cell–regenerative properties make it excellent for skin preparations. Rose oil is best known for its perfume and its effect on the spiritual aspects of the human psyche. It has a very delicate, sweet aroma, and is an excellent hormone balancer and leveller of mood swings.
Effects and uses	Circulatory: poor, sluggish circulation, haemorrhoids Excretory: cystitis Head: gingivitis, mouth ulcers Muscular: sprains Nervous: anxiety (panic), crying, depression, grief, hyperactivity, insecurity*, tantrums* Respiratory: asthma, bronchitis, common cold Skin: burns, chicken pox*, cuts, eczema, inflammation, rashes, ringworm*, scar tissue, shingles*, sunburn, wounds
Blends aromatically with	frankincense, geranium, mandarin, orange (sweet), sandalwood, ylang ylang
Cautions	None known

Common name   ROSEWOOD

Note   Base

Latin name   *Aniba rosaeodora*

Family   Lauraceae

Description   A tropical, medium-sized evergreen tree bearing yellow flowers with a reddish bark and wood, rosewood is native to the Amazon region and is used extensively for timber, although some goes to the Far East for the making of culinary equipment. The tree can grow up to 37 m (125 ft). In Brazil, for every tree cut down a new one must now be planted to preserve rosewood plantations and forests. The rose-scented wood chippings are steam distilled to yield a pale yellow essential oil with a very sweet floral woody aroma with spicy undertones.

General properties   A useful antiseptic for the skin and stimulating to the immune system when feeling low and under attack from infection. A good cell and tissue regenerator, rosewood oil is therefore helpful in the treatment of wounds and scars. Its cephalic and anticonvulsant properties are beneficial to a tired and uptight nervous system.

Effects and uses   Digestive: nausea*, travel sickness*
Immune system: stimulant*
Nervous: agitation, anxiety, depression
Reproductive: thrush (Candida)
Respiratory: bronchial infections, croup, hayfever*
Skin: acne, boils, dry flaky skin, impetigo*, scabies

Blends aromatically with   cedarwood, frankincense, geranium, ginger, lavender, sandalwood

Cautions   None known

Common name	SANDALWOOD
Note	Base
Latin name	*Santalum album*
Family	Santalaceae
Description	This fairly small (9 m/30 ft), elegant tree with slender branches, leathery leaves and light purple flowers attaches its roots to the roots of nearby trees and for the first seven years of its life derives most of its nourishment from the host tree. Sandalwood has been used for hundreds of years to make temple furniture; the Egyptians used it for many medicines and also embalming. The tree takes 30 years to mature before it can be used for its essential oil, which is obtained by steam distilling chippings of the heartwood and roots. A tree is planted each time one is cut down.
General properties	A nerve-relaxing base note, sandalwood is a good antiseptic, in particular for the respiratory system and urinary tract. Its astringent quality makes it effective for diarrhoea. Extensively used in the production of incense and as a fixative in cosmetics and aftershaves.
Effects and uses	Circulatory: chilblains*
	Digestive: abdominal pain (relaxant), diarrhoea, haemorrhoids, heartburn, travel sickness
	Excretory: bedwetting*, cystitis, urinary infections
	Nervous: anxiety*, depression, hyperactivity, insecurity, insomnia, neuralgia (nerve relaxant), tantrums
	Respiratory: bronchitis, catarrh, common cold, coughs, croup, sore throat, throat infections
	Skin: acne, cradle cap, dry eczema, dry skin, insect bites, nappy rash, rashes, sunburn
Blends aromatically with	bergamot, cypress, orange (sweet), rosemary, rose otto, rosewood
Cautions	None known

Common name	TEA TREE
Note	Top
Latin name	*Melaleuca alternifolia*
Family	Myrtaceae
Description	Tea tree is a small tree-shaped bush, native to the marshlands of Australia. Early European explorers are said to have infused the leaves to make a drink of tea – hence the name. Its small leaves are similar to those of the eucalyptus tree; the essential oil is found in tiny pockets in the leaf which release the oil when the leaf is snapped. Tea tree is a member of the Myrtaceae family, whose plants all bear their essential oils in the leaves or bark.
General properties	An exceptionally active but gentle oil, useful on many types of bacteria, fungi and viruses. Reputed to be stronger than many household antiseptics. An uplifting top note and a powerful stimulant to the immune system, tea tree oil is therefore extremely useful as a prophlylactic. It has a fresh, antiseptic-type odour and is used in toothpastes, gargles, disinfectants and aftershaves.
Effects and uses	Circulatory: haemorrhoids Digestive: threadworms, thrush Excretory: cystitis*, urinary infections Hair: dandruff, lice, nits Head: earache, gum infection, sinus troubles, teething, thrush Nervous: debility, depression Reproductive: genital infections, thrush (Candida) Respiratory: bronchitis, common cold, throat infections Skin: acne, athlete's foot, boils, cuts, impetigo, insect bites, ringworm, scabies
Blends aromatically with	geranium, lavender, lemon, marjoram (sweet)
Cautions	None known

Common name	THYME (SWEET)
Note	Top
Latin name	*Thymus vulgaris* (linalool or geraniol chemotypes)
Family	Lamiaceae
Description	There are dozens of different types of thyme, and the chemical composition varies from plant to plant, yielding several different thyme oils: sweet thymes, which are suitable for use on children, and red thymes (phenolic), with a characteristically powerful aroma – not suitable for children, but unfortunately the one most often found in shops on account of it being easily available commercially and also less expensive. The tiny dark green leaves form a very bushy ground-covering shrub. It flowers in late summer, producing pink/white flowers with tiny, very delicate petals. It is a highly aromatic plant used extensively in cooking to flavour meats and pasta.
General properties	Sweet thyme is effective against many types of viral and bacterial attacks, being a strong but gentle antiseptic. Its anti-inflammatory properties have a soothing effect on bronchitis and rheumatism. Its sweet, uplifting and energizing aroma is purifying and helpful against fatigue. Sweet thyme is a must for any sick room as it is an immuno-stimulant.
Effects and uses	Digestive: bad breath*, gum infections*, threadworms, thrush Excretory: cystitis, fluid retention, urinary infections Hair: lice, nits Head: earache (inflammation), gum infection, sinus troubles, sore throat, throat infection, tonsillitis Immune system: stimulant Nervous: anxiety, fatigue, hyperactivity, insomnia Respiratory: bronchial infections, bronchial spasm, common cold, coughs, croup Skin: infected acne, weeping eczema, psoriasis, ringworm, scabies, ulcers, verrucae, warts
Blends aromatically with	bergamot, lavender, lemon, rosemary
Cautions	None known

Common name	YLANG YLANG
Note	Base
Latin name	*Cananga odorata*
Family	Anonaceae
Description	Native to the Philippines, now grown in Madagascar, the cananga tree can grow to 20 m (65 ft) in height, although trees grown for essential oils are pruned to an accessible height. When the flowers first form they are green and hairy; 20 days later the fully formed flowers are deep yellow and bell shaped, and are picked before 10 a.m. to get the best oil. They are steam distilled immediately to prevent the petals from spoiling. The trees grow in rich volcanic soil in moist tropical conditions. Ylang ylang oil is used extensively as a fixative in expensive perfumes.
General properties	Ylang ylang is renowned for its aphrodisiac qualities. It has soothing properties on the nerves and is a sedative. It has antiseptic effects and is especially calming on erratic breathing. It was thought to be stimulating to the scalp in Victorian times, when it was used in a hair preparation known as 'Macassar' (which left oily marks on furniture – hence the need for an 'anti-macassar', a cover to protect the backs of arm chairs).
Effects and uses	Digestive: colic (antispasmodic), diabetes, intestinal infections Hair: scalp tonic, thinning hair Nervous: anxiety, crying, hyperactivity, insecurity[*], insomnia, nightmares, tantrums Respiratory: rapid, deep breathing (hyperpnoea) Skin: oily skin
Blends aromatically with	chamomile (Roman), lavender, rose otto
Cautions	None known

Expressed Oils

Common name	BERGAMOT
Note	Top
Latin name	*Citrus bergamia*
Family	Rutaceae
Description	The fruit takes its name from a small town in northern Italy where it was first traded. The bergamot tree is a member of the Rutaceae family and bears small, pitted orange-like fruit. The tree grows up to 4.5 m (15 ft) in height and has long, smooth oval-shaped leaves. The essential oil is stored in the same way as with all the other citrus fruits – in tiny pockets in the peel – and is obtained by expression. Bergamot oil is used to impart the delicate perfumed flavour to Earl Grey tea, the recipe of which was given to the second Earl Grey by an envoy from China.
General properties	This uplifting top note oil has soothing and antiseptic qualities useful for skin conditions, especially if they are stress related. Bergamot is an excellent tonic for the digestive system and is active against cold sores. The oil is pale yellow/green in colour and has a fresh, light, fruity aroma with a hint of spice.
Effects and uses	Digestive: colic, flatulence, indigestion, loss of appetite, nausea, travel sickness Head: mouth ulcers (oral thrush) Nervous: agitation, anxiety, apathy, depression, hyperactivity, insomnia Respiratory: common cold Skin: allergies*, cold sores, dermatitis, eczema, psoriasis, ulcers, verrucae, warts, wounds (*see caution below*)
Blends aromatically with	cedarwood, chamomile (Roman), cypress, geranium, lavender, mandarin, marjoram (sweet), sandalwood, thyme (sweet)
Cautions	Not to be used undiluted; as the oil is a photosensitizer it should always be diluted and there should be no exposure to sunlight or UV light until at least an hour after its use

Common name   LEMON
Note   Top
Latin name   *Citrus limon*
Family   Rutaceae
Description   This tree is similar in bearing to the orange tree except that it bears stiff thorns and the leaves are serrated. The lemons tend not always to be exactly the same shape as the lemons you see in the supermarket because they are not treated with sprays or chemicals. The essential oil is expressed from tiny pockets in the skin and smells like the fruit. This member of the Rutaceae family is a native of Asia, but now can be found growing wild in Mediterranean regions.
General properties   The fresh, juicy aroma of this essential oil is uplifting to the spirit and is a general all-round tonic. Its gentle antiseptic and antimicrobial action helps maintain a healthy palate and digestion. Lemon oil stimulates the production of white corpuscles and thus helps the body to fight off infection.
Effects and uses   Circulatory: anaemia, chilblains, cold feet, fluid retention, poor circulation, thread veins
Digestive: diabetes, diarrhoea, flatulence, gastro-enteritis, jaundice (liver tonic), loss of appetite, nausea, round worms, sluggish digestion, travel sickness
Hair: greasy dandruff, seborrhoea of scalp
Head: headaches, nosebleeds, oral thrush
Immune system: stimulant
Muscular: rheumatism (anti-inflammatory)
Nervous: insomnia, nightmares, sluggishness (invigorating)
Respiratory: air antiseptic, common cold, influenza
Skin: boils, broken capillaries, bruises, chicken pox*, greasy skin, insect bites, measles*, verrucae, warts
Blends aromatically with   cypress, eucalyptus, geranium, ginger, lavender, orange (sweet), tea tree, thyme (sweet)
Cautions   Not to be used undiluted; as the oil is a mild photosensitizer it should always be diluted and there should be no exposure to sunlight or UV light until at least an hour after its use

Common name	MANDARIN
Note	Top
Latin name	*Citrus reticulata*
Family	Rutaceae
Description	An evergreen tree with small glossy leaves, native to China and the Far East, *C. reticulata* bears small fragrant flowers and very sweet, fleshy fruit. First brought to Europe in the 19th century and then to the US (where it was re-named tangerine and developed to a larger size). The original fruit was given to the noble Mandarins of China as a gift. The tree grows to a height of 6 m (20 ft) and the oil is obtained by expression from tiny pockets in the peel.
General properties	This top note essential oil has a sweet floral aroma and is calming to the nervous system. Its best-known actions are on the digestive system, being a very mild laxative and general tonic to this system, as well as stimulant to the liver. It also soothes abdominal pain.
Effects and uses	Digestive: abdominal pain, colic, constipation, heartburn, hiccoughs[*], indigestion, liver tonic, nausea, stomach cramp Nervous: anxiety, excitability, hyperactivity, insomnia, moodiness, tantrums
Blends aromatically with	bergamot, chamomile (Roman), rose otto
Cautions	Not to be used undiluted, as the oil is a slight photosensitizer

Common name	ORANGE (SWEET)
Note	Top
Latin name	*Citrus aurantium* var. *sinensis*
Family	Rutaceae
Description	This member of the Rutaceae family is native to China and bears small fleshy fruit. The tree itself is much smaller than the bitter orange tree. The essential oil is expressed from tiny pockets in the peel to give a sweet, fresh fruity smell. The Crusaders are thought to have brought the orange to Europe, as it was certainly available in the 16th century. The ancient Chinese used to dry the peel and use it for herbal tinctures and medicines.
General properties	Essence of sweet orange has been used for years in cooking, especially in rich fruit cakes – this may be due to its excellent action on the digestive system. Its calming properties make this oil especially useful for nervous disorders. A very balancing oil, which raises the spirits.
Effects and uses	Digestive: constipation, indigestion, gastro-enteritis, mild liver tonic, nausea, travel sickness Head: mouth ulcers Nervous: anxiety, nervousness, vertigo
Blends aromatically with	frankincense, ginger, lemon, rose otto, sandalwood
Cautions	Not to be used neat, as the oil is a slight photosensitizer

N.B. Properties and effects of the 20 chosen oils have been taken from:
Franchomme P, Pénoël D 1990 *L'Aromathérapie Exactement*. Jollois, Limoges
Price S, Price L 1999 *Aromatherapy for Health Professionals*. Churchill Livingstone, London

Storing Your Oils

Essential oils should always be stored in dark brown glass bottles and kept away from strong sunlight and other strong smells. Ideally, they should be stored at a temperature of 15 – 20°C (59 –68°F) and the caps should always be firmly in place to prevent loss through evaporation. Keep all essential oils away from heat and safely away from animals and children. The best place is on the top shelf of a high cupboard in the bathroom or kitchen.

Always ensure that the essential oils you buy have droppers fitted in the bottles. This is a safety precaution and ensures that if a child does get hold of a bottle of essential oil he is unlikely to swallow the whole bottle-full because only one drop comes out at a time. Essential oils taste horrible when they are undiluted, so a child is unlikely to try more than one drop!

Essential oils should always be kept away from the eyes, the genital area and other mucous membranes unless used under the guidance of an aromatherapist who belongs to a professional aromatherapy association.

When you have made your own blends, keep them in dark glass bottles with a label and with the cap tightly screwed on. Your mixture should last from six to nine months if stored correctly. Oils blended with carriers do not need to have a dropper in the bottle; however it is still advisable to keep them well out of reach of children. Although correctly diluted oils do not present a hazard, it is better not to let anybody in your household who is not familiar with aromatherapy use your own personal mixtures.

Purity and Quality

To obtain the best results from your aromatherapy treatments you must endeavour to buy the best quality essential oils that are available – the best will be from a specialist supplier. A good quality essential oil will be available in a dark brown or black glass bottle. Some come in pretty blue bottles, but these are not as light-resistant as brown ones. The label must have not only the common name of the essential oil but also its Latin name – and sometimes the variety of the plant. The label should also contain warnings about keeping the oils out of reach of children and animals and away from the eyes.

The aroma of a good quality essential oil will be strong and vigorous. Organic oils or oils which are the product of natural farming methods are obviously the best because of the complete absence of unwanted chemicals such as pesticides or artificial fertilizers; it is also possible to obtain such oils from wild plants. The aroma of the best quality essential oils varies naturally from year to year because of environmental changes in weather and soil conditions.

Always buy your oils from a reputable and knowledgeable company. Many of the oils mentioned in this chapter are specific to their Latin names, for instance *Eucalyptus smithii*, which is a particular type of eucalyptus safe for use on children. There are other types of eucalyptus (such as *E. globulus* or *E. radiata*) which are not quite as safe as *E. smithii* when used on the skin, therefore buy a bottle with a label that states exactly what is inside, not merely 'eucalyptus'. Marjoram also comes into this category, as Spanish marjoram (*Thymus mastichina*) has different constituents from sweet marjoram (*Origanum majorana*).

Good quality oils do not come cheap; however, just because you have paid a lot for your oil do not assume that it is of high quality – remember only that a good quality oil is not available at a cheap price. The importance of using a good quality oil will be obvious once you see its healing effects on your child. Some essential oils may have synthetics or other chemicals added to dilute or stretch them. The presence of synthetic molecules in an essential oil will interfere with its natural synergy and consequently the oil's healing properties, therefore choosing an essential oil for its purity is a must. Essential oils which contain synthetic molecules or which have been diluted may well irritate your child's skin or cause other problems, therefore it cannot be stressed too strongly that quality and purity are paramount when looking to essential oils to maintain or improve the health of your children. (*See Useful Addresses.*)

Precautions

Essential oils are very powerful and should only be used in small doses. When you are using essential oils, follow these guidelines:

1 If your child becomes suddenly ill with something you do not understand, take him immediately to a doctor and do not attempt to diagnose and treat the child yourself at home.

2 Do not attempt to replace your child's existing medication unless under the guidance of your GP and an aromatherapist or aromatologist.

3 Should you be at all undecided about which oils to use on your child, consult a qualified aromatherapist who will help and guide you in the right direction.

4 Keep the oils away from your child's eyes, being careful when massaging the back of their hands not to let your child rub the oils into his eyes. Should any essential oils get into the eyes, wash it out with a pure vegetable carrier oil before seeking medical advice.

5 Do not use vaporizers which have a naked flame in the form of a candle, which might be knocked over accidentally.

6 Never take essential oils by mouth unless under the guidance of a suitably qualified practitioner, such as an aromatologist, ideally working in cooperation with your own doctor.

7 If your child is taking homoeopathic remedies, the essential oil treatments must be given at a different time of day to prevent them interfering with the homoeopathic treatment.

8 Store all essential oils in dark brown glass bottles in a cool dark place out of reach of children.

9 Stick only to recommended doses. Do not attempt to go above the recommended dosage unless under the guidance of a qualified aromatherapist or aromatologist.

10 Always use high quality essential oils identified by the botanical name and giving the chemical variety of the oil where appropriate. For example, *Thymus vulgaris* is the botanical name for thyme. It is possible to buy a very powerful, and much cheaper, thyme containing phenols, but a sweet thyme containing gentle alcohols is much to be preferred for use on children, as it is hazard-free. Buy only from a reputable recommended source where there is a qualified person who can give you advice.

11 Finally, make sure that every mixture you make up has a label telling you exactly what is in it, what you are using it for and the date the mixture was made. This prevents confusion when treating different children and ailments.

3

Different Carriers, Their Properties and Their Uses

A carrier is anything which can 'carry' essential oils into the body, for example air, water, lotion, cream – plus those used for massage, namely fixed and macerated vegetable oils.

There are many different carriers that can be used in aromatherapy; these include honey, milk and shampoo, all of which are discussed in Chapter 4. There are also one or two substances which should not be used, such as animal fat and mineral oils – and we will discuss these first.

1) Mineral Oil

Mineral oil, which is used as baby oil because of its non-penetrating quality, is in fact not a very good medium for essential oils. This is because mineral oil forms a barrier on the surface of the skin to prevent moisture getting in or out. This barrier is essential when wanting to prevent baby's urine from having an adverse effect on the skin, but it would also hinder the essential oils from passing easily through the skin and into the bloodstream to act upon the body.

2) Animal Fat

An animal fat commonly used on the skin is lanolin, which is a fat derived from sheep's wool – and used frequently in cosmetics. Like mineral oil, it is composed of large molecules and forms a barrier over the skin. It is not suitable for use with essential oils, as it can impede their passage. Unfortunately the large lanolin molecules can also increase the size of the pore openings on the skin of the face (and body), so strictly speaking it is not suitable even for cosmetic use.

Before discussing the qualities and properties of carriers which *can* be applied to the body (such as vegetable oils and emulsified lotion), let us look at two carriers which are often used as a method of getting essential oils into the body.

Air

Air is not often thought of as a 'carrier' (except, perhaps in relation to infectious diseases!). However, essential oil molecules, 'carried' in the air, can be inhaled easily.

Inhalation is the quickest treatment method since the oils can be inhaled directly into the bloodstream via the lungs. Because of this benefit, and because of the psychological benefits of inhalation, air is a very useful and versatile carrier (*see Chapter 4*). In fact, whichever method you may use with your essential oils, air will also be involved to some extent as a carrier.

Perhaps it is prudent to mention here that however efficient air is as a carrier, and however genuine are your oils, obvious pollutants such as cigarette smoke, etc. should be avoided. Neither is it a good idea to add your essential oils to the pot-pourri normally available, as most of these are fragranced already with synthetic aromas (you should try to buy unfragranced pot-pourri to which you can then add your essential oils).

Water

Although water is an excellent carrier for baths, compresses, vaporizers, hair rinses and gargles, essential oils do not usually mix well with water, so remember always to shake a blend of water and essential oils very well before use. (For methods of using essential oils with water, *see Chapter 4*.)

Any water used should not have any obvious pollutants or synthetic detergents in it.

Carriers for Application and Massage

Lotion, cream and vegetable oil carriers are used to dilute and spread essential oils over the body to enable them to be absorbed evenly by the skin.

If we are to take the time and trouble to find the best quality essential oils possible, then it is absolutely essential that we should also be looking for quality carrier bases in which to put them. It is of little use if the majority of the aromatherapy treatment (97 per cent carrier) is of such poor quality that it impairs the therapeutic benefits of the true essential oil.

Lotion Carrier

Sometimes we do not need to 'massage' an area of the body to achieve a good result – often only simple direct application is required. For this a bland vegetable-based lotion is much more useful as a carrier than a vegetable oil. A lotion has several advantages over a vegetable oil for everyday use on children:

1 It is lighter to use, as it is non-greasy and readily absorbed into the skin.
2 It is cleaner to apply as it does not leave an oily residue on the hands, or subsequently on the bottle.
3 Even when applied several times daily, lotion does not stain the skin or the clothes.
4 If the lotion is accidentally tipped over, it is less likely to flood out and make a mess. If it does spill, it is much easier to clean up than oil.
5 Lotion is cooling and is to be preferred as a carrier on conditions like sunburn, inflammation, insect bites, feverish conditions (chicken pox, measles), flu, etc.
6 Because it is an emulsion, carrier lotion will mix evenly in the bath water and, in our opinion, is a safer and more effective way of using oils in the bath for children. Use the chart in Chapter 4 (*see page 65*) for the number of drops of essential oil to be added to 50 ml of lotion, and the method of use.
7 Carrier lotion is a perfect base to which to add up to 15 per cent of a specialized or macerated carrier oil to enrich its qualities; this makes it a very versatile medium for home treatment (*see Chapter 4*).

Cream Carrier

To use a cream as a carrier, you must first be sure that it is not perfumed or containing synthetic molecules. Since most of us are not chemists, we suggest you buy base creams (and lotions) from a reputable aromatherapy company (*see Useful Addresses*).

Creams are very useful carriers for use on small areas (such as the face, hands, feet, knees, elbows, etc.) where the skin may be very dry, chapped or cracked.

Vegetable Carrier Oils

Although not so acceptable for application purposes, vegetable oils are indispensable for massage because they take a little while to penetrate; thus the skin remains smooth and the hands can move easily over it. Also, although vegetable oils cannot penetrate the skin and access the bloodstream to the same extent as essential oils (because the molecules are too large), they are very nourishing to the top layers of the skin and benefit this part of the body. As we know, vegetable oils are edible and, to benefit from the properties of the larger molecules, the oils have to be used in or on food (as olive oil on salads) or in capsules (for example, evening primrose oil, garlic oil).

Vegetable oils are what we call 'fixed' oils, which simply means that they are not volatile – in other words they do not evaporate when exposed to the air (unlike essential oils). A simple test can be done to prove this: if you drop one drop of essential oil onto a piece of blotting paper the mark will disappear quite quickly (within a few days), leaving no trace (save any colour, if present). However, if you place a drop of carrier oil onto a piece of blotting paper, the translucent stain will remain virtually for ever.

For aromatherapy we use only 'fixed' vegetable oils which are cold pressed, for example sunflower or almond, as carriers. Animals fats and mineral oils are never used.

The term 'cold pressed' applies to many of the fixed oils we are going to discuss in this chapter. Cold pressing is an extraction process in which no solvents have been used and no heat applied (which can interfere with the quality and purity of a carrier oil). The remaining pulp is sent for animal food or to a factory where much more oil can be extracted by processing it with solvents and steam, which produces a less expensive oil for commercial use.

The terms 'virgin' and 'extra virgin' apply only to olive oil. Extra virgin refers to the first pressing of the olives, virgin to the second pressing. Usually the darker the olive oil, the more likely it is to be the product of a first or second pressing.

Buying Vegetable Carrier Oils

Unfortunately, buying a pure carrier oil is not as easy as you might think. Although cold-pressed oils are available from aromatherapy suppliers and some health food shops, they can be difficult to find in a supermarket (except for virgin olive oils). Also, even cold-pressed avocado and macadamia oils are often sent to a chemical refining plant to be decolourized and deodorized, as these treatments are believed to make them more cosmetically acceptable. Take care when buying from a chemist, as most oils stocked by chemists will be refined. These are not appropriate for aromatherapy.

When you go round the supermarket for the weekly shopping and are faced with a vast array of different cooking oils on the shelves, do not be misled into thinking that these oils are exactly the same as an aromatherapist would use as a carrier – they are not. The majority of oils on supermarket shelves have been treated chemically – that is, taken from the plant material with solvents, then stabilized and purified. They are stabilized to take them up to high temperatures so that food such as chips, etc. can be cooked without the oil breaking down; they are 'purified' (that is, bleached and recoloured) to ensure standardization on the shelves.

There are, however, a few cold-pressed oils which are available from the supermarket. Unfortunately cold pressing is a much more expensive process and therefore these oils are less readily available and more expensive. Sometimes a manufacturer may put a 'cold-pressed' label onto a poor quality oil; however, you can have some idea of what to buy by considering the following factors:

1 The richer the colour of the oil, depending on the plant origin, the more likely it is that the oil has not been chemically refined. The deeper colour and a slight aroma should indicate that the vegetable oil is of a higher quality, though sometimes cold-pressed vegetable oils are de-colourized and then recoloured to keep the colour standard (those from an aromatherapy supplier may vary slightly in colour from harvest to harvest, as do essential oils).
2 Check the sell-by date. If an oil is unrefined it will only last six to nine months at the most in bright light. A highly refined oil (which may be labelled 'pure' simply because it has been chemically purified), although not so good for aromatherapy, will last much longer.

Maceration

This method is usually used on plants that cannot be steam distilled for commercial and/or practical reasons. There are a few plants from which it is very expensive to extract essential oils by distillation, as the percentage of oil within them is very small. To extract the health-giving properties from such plants, for example calendula, the flowerheads are collected and placed in a base vegetable oil such as sunflower or almond (preferably organically grown). This mixture is left in a warm place for several days, being stirred frequently till the base carrier oil has absorbed the volatile essential oil plus any other properties from the plant material which are soluble in the base vegetable oil. A small amount of natural preservative (such as wheatgerm oil which contains vitamin E) is then added. This process is called maceration and the end result resembles, in effect, a weak ready-mixed massage oil, each one having its own special benefits to the skin and/or the body.

Macerated oils can be used either on their own (for extra therapeutic effects) or in a dilution of 25 – 50 per cent in a lighter base oil such as sunflower, almond, jojoba or grapeseed. The amount of essential oil already present in a macerated oil is very slight but effective, and drops of selected essential oils can also be added in the normal manner to increase the therapeutic effect of the mix. If diluting a macerated oil in another carrier base, there will only be a minute amount of its essential oil and other therapeutic properties present in your total carrier oil, therefore you should add the normal recommended number of drops of pure essential oils to get the maximum benefit from your treatments.

Macerated oils, in their own right, are beneficial not only to the skin but also to the rest of the body, because their own molecules of essential oil can access the bloodstream.

It can be quite interesting to make your own macerated oil. Look around your garden and see if you have any aromatic plants such as lavender, sage, rosemary, honeysuckle (from which no essential oil is available) or rose. Fill a 1-kg (2-lb) glass jar three-quarters full with organic sunflower oil and one teaspoonful of wheatgerm oil. Take the flowers and/or leaves that you wish to macerate, and add them to the jar of oil till it is full. Put the lid on tightly and leave the jar in a sunny place; if there is not much sunshine to be had, a warm place like the airing cupboard is ideal. Shake on a daily basis and, after one week, use a sieve to separate the oil from the flower material. If you feel that the resultant oil is not strongly scented enough for you, you may add fresh plant material to your oil and repeat the process for a further week.

Storing Cold-pressed and Macerated Oils

Unfortunately, because the best vegetable carrier oils used in aromatherapy are unrefined, they can become rancid quite quickly due to oxidization, especially if they are not stored properly. Although they are not often found in dark glass bottles, keeping them in this way protects the oils from deterioration by light. However, whether they are bought in dark glass, clear glass or plastic bottles, unrefined, cold-pressed and macerated oils should always be kept in a cool, dark cupboard away from any heat, as they easily deteriorate when exposed to warmth and light.

The top should be screwed on tightly so that air is not allowed to enter the bottle. Another tip is to decant the oil into a smaller bottle as it is used up, as the less air present in the bottle, the slower the rate of oxidization and therefore the slower the onset of rancidity.

Conclusion

Cold-pressed, unrefined oils are much better not only for aromatherapy, but for the family's diet, as these oils are whole and have not been interfered with in the same manner as a chemically treated oil. Since much of today's modern illness is caused by preservatives, stabilizers and junk food, it makes sense to look for these oils anyway to enable the health of your family to be improved from the inside out.

Unfortunately, these oils do cost a little more money; however, in our opinion, this is well worth it. Who can put a price on health?

In the sample recipes in Chapter 5 we illustrate the versatility of a small range of carrier oils that can limit the cost of a basic aromatherapy kit for home use. However, in this chapter we include a few more so that you can make your own choice from among the carrier oils available.

We are now going to look at the individual properties of the two distinctly different types of carrier oils (pure vegetable and macerated).

For more information – and a further selection of carrier oils, see *Aromatherapy Workbook* and *Aromatherapy Carrier Oils* (details in the Bibliography).

Vegetable Carrier Oils

Almond Oil
Cold-pressed sweet almond oil is a pretty pale yellow colour with little odour (the refined oil has none) and a hint of marzipan in the flavour. It contains vitamins in its chemical make-up, including vitamin E, and has less tendency to become rancid, lasting up to 18 months without added preservatives provided it is stored as recommended above. Almond oil is quite oily and it is often recommended to be used in dilution with a finer carrier oil such as sunflower or grapeseed.

It is an excellent emollient oil, alleviating dry skin and nourishing it; it also helps to soothe inflammation. Almond oil is beneficial in relieving the itching caused by eczema, psoriasis and dermatitis and all cases of dry scaly skin. Because it is slightly thicker than grapeseed or sunflower oils, it will take slightly longer to be absorbed into the skin's layers, thus helping very dry skin against water loss for a longer period of time.

Avocado Oil
Avocado oil is pressed from fruits which are too ripe to be sold at the market. These fruits are sliced and dried in the sun (quite a long, tedious affair) before being cold pressed. The resultant oil is thick and occasionally may have residues of avocado flesh, making it slightly cloudy if kept in conditions that are too cold. This can be a good sign, showing that the avocado oil has been cold pressed and untampered with (the cloudiness will clear if the oil is placed in a warm place for a few minutes).

Avocado oil is a deep green colour and contains vitamins A, B and D. It has excellent keeping qualities and is quite a thick oil, normally being diluted with a finer carrier oil like grapeseed or sunflower in up to 25 per cent dilution. Refined avocado oil bought from a chemist or health food store is a pale yellowy green and is not recommended for therapeutic use.

Avocado oil is very penetrating, with skin-healing properties. and is very valuable for massage when treating dry skin conditions, which would indicate its use for dry eczema and psoriasis. It is a beneficial oil to add to your basic carrier if your child is overweight, because of its good penetration.

Avocado oil, if taken, is easily digested and can be helpful in treating gastric problems and constipation.

Grapeseed Oil

Grapeseed oil is usually produced in France alongside the wine industry. The grapes are used to make the wine and the wasted grape seeds are washed and dried. Grape seeds cannot be pressed, so unfortunately heat has to be applied during extraction methods. A large aromatherapy firm (*see Useful Addresses*) can sometimes ask for the oil to be 'rescued' before it is taken to a chemical refining plant to be decolourized, deodorized and recoloured. The grapeseed oil used in aromatherapy should be that which has not been refined after extraction. The oil is almost odourless and contains vitamins E and F. Oil which has not been refined is a pale yellowy-green.

Grapeseed can be used on its own in a massage preparation, as it is very light and fine on the skin. It is especially useful for children who have greasy skin. It is hypoallergenic, therefore makes a perfect base oil to use on children prone to allergic reactions.

Used as a food, it is easy to digest and is useful for hypertension.

Hazelnut Oil

Hazelnut is a lovely, light, yellow-brown oil cold pressed from the nut. It has a characteristic odour which should blend favourably with your chosen essential oils. If desired, it can be diluted with 50 per cent sunflower or grapeseed.

Hazelnut oil is beneficial for greasy skin as it helps to dissolve sebum; it is astringent. Circulatory problems can also be helped by hazelnut, as it is stimulating to this system.

The unrefined oil is delicious on salads.

Olive Oil

Olive oil, like avocado, is obtained from the flesh of the fruit. It is a deep-green colour and has a characteristic odour which is not always acceptable to children and may overpower the smell of your essential oils. Although rather thick, it can be diluted up to 75 per cent with a lighter carrier such as grapeseed or sunflower. It is very stable and can usually last 18 months without the addition of stabilizers.

Olive oil has the properties of being calming to the skin and is very emollient, leaving a silky smooth feel which may be termed greasy by those who do not have a dry skin. It relieves itching and can be used on insect bites, burns, bruises and sprains. It is helpful in getting rid of dandruff or cradle cap, especially if mixed with rosemary essential oil.

Used in or on food, olive oil has a reputation for lowering blood cholesterol levels better than a fatless diet.

Rose Hip Oil

Rose hip oil is usually extracted from wild or organically grown rose hips. It is a lovely golden colour but, like grapeseed oil, cannot be extracted by cold pressing and has to be treated with steam. As it is not a commercially produced oil, it is not refined after extraction. It has a high percentage of vitamin C.

Rose hip oil is regenerative to the skin, so is most beneficial for scar tissue, wounds, burns, sunburn, dermatitis, eczema and psoriasis. Mothers will be interested to know that it is also an oil which can delay the signs of ageing if used regularly.

Sunflower Oil

Most sunflower oil on the supermarket shelves is solvent extracted and is therefore not appropriate for aromatherapy; however, cold-pressed sunflower oil is available from some aromatherapy suppliers. This oil has a lovely, light, non-greasy feel to it, leaving the skin feeling satiny smooth; it can be used as a base on its own and also as a diluent for the heavier carrier oils. It contains vitamins A, D and E (mainly E).

Sunflower oil has a prophylactic effect on the skin, making it beneficial for bruises and other skin problems such as ulcers (especially leg ulcers). It also helps circulatory problems.

Used on or in food, sunflower oil helps to maintain healthy teeth in children.[1] Sunflower seeds (therefore the oil also) are reputedly beneficial for asthmatics (traditionally the flowers have been used against many different types of chest problems).[2]

Wheatgerm Oil

Wheatgerm oil is a deep orange-brown colour and is cold pressed from the germ of the wheat. It is a very thick oil which is usually diluted up to 75 per cent in a lighter base oil such as sunflower or grapeseed. Wheatgerm oil is a natural preservative and a small amount can be added to other oils to give them a longer life. This preservation property is due to wheatgerm's high vitamin E content.

Wheatgerm can be rather heavy for very small children and its use is recommended only on children over six years old. Take care in use, as if used in too high a percentage, the wheatgerm oil will stain your towels and clothing.

It is effective on dry skin (as in eczema); when taken in or on food it is good for indigestion and also helps maintain healthy spines, bones and muscle tissue in growing children. This may be particularly helpful for girls with Rett Syndrome.[3]

Macerated Carrier Oils

Calendula

To obtain this lovely orange-yellow oil, the flowerheads are macerated in almond or sunflower oil (we use organically grown flowers and organic sunflower oil).

Calendula oil can be used successfully in cases of nappy rash, bruises, cuts and grazes, skin abscesses, eczema, psoriasis and dry, chapped skin. It is anti-inflammatory and a tonic to the circulatory system, being astringent, and also helpful against varicose veins and broken veins.

Internally, it has been used for indigestion and period problems such as painful or scanty menstruation.[1]

Carrot Oil

Macerated carrot oil is a lovely orange colour and contains vitamins A, B, C, D, E and F. It is usually macerated in sunflower seed oil and needs a lot of attention and care in the process. Care is needed not to confuse macerated carrot oil with the extract beta-carotene (often sold as carrot oil), which is a very deep orange and which will stain the skin.

Carrot oil has marvellous anti-inflammatory and anti-irritant effects and is useful on all insect bites, sprains, eczema, psoriasis; it is often used in sun preparations and is of help in healing scar tissue. Mothers will be interested to know that, used regularly, carrot oil delays the signs of ageing.

Hypericum

Hypericum, commonly known as St John's wort, is a deep red macerated oil. The plant has yellow flowers and buds, the deep red colour of the oil coming from the buds (try squeezing one between your fingers). It is a most useful oil therapeutically, both externally and internally.

Hypericum oil is soothing, antiseptic and analgesic (pain-relieving) on the skin, making it perfect for relieving insect bites, open sores, bruises or wounds and also rheumatic pain. It can be used to soothe sunburn – also nerve inflammation (for example, neuralgia) or nerve tissue damage. It is frequently used against burns, as it lowers the skin temperature.

Hypericum is beneficial for bedwetting when massaged into the lower back, especially with the addition of essential oils (cypress, rosemary).

This versatile oil is also beneficial for depression – and, used in or on food, for gastritis.[4]

Lime Blossom Oil

Macerated lime blossom oil is a beautiful pale yellow oil which blends very well with essential oils.

The oil is soothing for aches and pains and is useful for both insomnia and stress.

1 Price L 1999 *Carrier Oils for Aromatherapy and Massage.* Riverhead, Stratford–upon–Avon
2 Price S 1993 *Aromatherapy Workbook.* Thorsons, London
3 Rett Syndrome is a rare neurological disorder which affects only girls (approximately 1 in 15,000). The symptoms usually begin to show themselves between nine and 18 months of age, before which time development is normal. Some of the many symptoms include reduced mobility, loss of purposeful use of the hands, very poor circulation in the lower limbs, incontinence, severe learning difficulties and (as the disorder progresses) curvature of the spine.
4 Mabey R 1988 *The Complete New Herbal.* Gaia Books Ltd, London

4

Methods of Using Essential Oils

Aromatherapists use essential oils to give professional treatments for all sorts of problems, both physical and mental; however, the oils can also be used very successfully at home for your family. Since this book is intended for non-professional use, the methods described in this chapter are just for home treatment. Should any other problems arise which you do not know how to treat, please consult a suitably qualified aromatherapist.

Since everyone is different and has different likes and dislikes, not all oils will be suitable for all people or for all their problems. This is especially true for children, who need to build up their likes and dislikes of different things as they travel through life. Always bear this in mind when treating your children, because the more they like an oil the more it is likely to work. A child who does not like your choice of oil may harbour negative feelings about essential oils and aromatherapy treatments as he gets older.

Inhalation

Inhalation is one of the most effective ways to use pure essential oils in aromatherapy. Indeed, the word aromatherapy means 'a treatment using smells', and what better way to use a smell than to 'sniff it with meaning'? Inhalation is also the quickest way that the essential oils can affect both body and mind, since when we inhale air it goes directly not only to the brain, which acts on the aroma molecules received, but also into the bloodstream via our lungs. Aromatherapy used this way can be instantly effective because when we inhale the vapours of an essential oil they are immediately in our system – going straight to work on our problems.

There are many ways by which we can inhale essential oils:

1) Vaporizers

By using a vaporizer we can spread essential oil (by evaporation of the molecules) throughout an entire space or area. This makes the essential oil beneficial not only to the child concerned but also to everybody else in the room. A vaporizer can be used not just for sickness but also to fragrance a room or to change the mood of any children within it. For example, a top note oil such as sweet orange or lemon is known to be uplifting to all who inhale it, whereas an oil such as ylang ylang or sandalwood is more sedative and relaxing (useful if the children at your child's party are getting too excited!).

Vaporizers are most often used in the sickroom, where essential oil vapour in the air can prevent the spread of infection. Many different common ailments can be treated by vaporization – for example asthma, coughs and colds, breathing difficulties, depression, insomnia and fatigue.

a) Candle Vaporizer/Burners

Candle vaporizers are very attractive but must be used properly and correctly to ensure safety at all times. In a candle vaporizer you will find a well in the top for water. It is important that this well is filled with water *before* you add the drops of essential oil or light the candle. When using essential oils in a vaporizer like this, four drops is sufficient to provide an effective treatment or to fragrance a whole room. Always make sure that it is well out of the reach of children because of the naked flame – and kept well away from other flammable substances.

b) Electric Vaporizers

Electric vaporizers do not need water added to them. The essential oils can be dropped directly into the top of the vaporizer, again using four drops. Where there are children running round a room an electric vaporizer is much safer than a candle burner/vaporizer for obvious reasons – and can be used in the same situations. Always follow the manufacturer's instructions for use.

2) On a Tissue

One or two drops of essential oil can be put on a tissue for a child to sniff whenever necessary. This method is used for nervous tension, colds, coughs and other airborne infections. Inhaling deeply from a tissue is helpful too for asthma sufferers when they have breathing difficulties. It can also be used for vertigo and travel sickness. With this method the child only takes a sniff of the essential oil when it is needed. Insomnia can be helped by placing the tissue (with the two drops of essential oil) just under the child's pillow slip, near his face. This way there is no chance of the essential oil getting in the child's eyes or onto his skin – it releases just enough essential oil to create a pleasant fragrance around the child's head.

This is possibly one of the best ways of introducing aromatherapy to new babies. If, after the baby is born, you put two drops of essential oil on a tissue and always keep it near you when you are feeding him, he will become accustomed to the aroma – and associate it with love, comfort and mummy. In this way he can be helped to sleep at night by placing the same aroma near him in the cot to reassure him that you are nearby. It also makes it much easier when you are leaving your baby with a babysitter – she too can have the same aroma with her so that, should your baby wake, he can be comforted by the same smell he has come to associate with contentment and pleasure.

3) On Cotton Wool

Four drops of essential oil on a cotton wool ball tucked behind a warm radiator will create the same effect as a vaporizer, as warm air from the radiator will evaporate the essential oil, creating a pleasant fragrance throughout the room.

4) Inhaling from Water

To relieve catarrh and nasal congestion, place one or two drops only of your chosen essential oil into a bowl of warm (not boiling) water. The child can then inhale the steam carrying the essential oil to help loosen the catarrh or relieve the congestion.

N.B. Never leave your child alone to do this.

Caution: The effect of the steam on an asthmatic child may worsen already difficult breathing; it may be preferable to let such a child breathe from a tissue.

Case Histories

(For reasons of confidentiality, all names have been changed.)

When Colin was two years old he was diagnosed as asthmatic. He had a history of chest infections, coughs, colds and sickness. His parents were advised to buy a nebulizer, which they did.

Not wanting Colin to be dependent later on in life on steroid inhalers, his mother, an aromatherapist, put 2 drops lavender and 2 drops *Eucalyptus smithii* on a tissue every evening and slipped it under Colin's pillowcase.

The night-time coughing improved almost immediately and, by using the same mixture in a vaporizer during the day alongside the nebulizer, the condition continued to improve. Colin is now becoming more stable – and with his sleep pattern improved, he is less irritable during the day, which leads to fewer attacks. The number of chest infections he has suffered has fallen dramatically over the last seven months.

The pleasant 'side-effect' is that because Colin sleeps all night so does everyone else, making family life much less fraught!

When one of Christine's children, Kevin, came home from school with a very heavy cold, she was naturally concerned – Kevin is one of seven children! Obviously, apart from helping Kevin it was important that she try and halt the spread of this viral infection to other members of her family.

It was decided to blend sweet thyme, *Eucalyptus smithii*, lemon and tea tree (1 ml of each) together in a small dropper bottle. Christine used 3 – 4 drops of this mixture on several tissues, tucking one behind each radiator in the house (the central heating was on). In Kevin's bedroom, which he shared with two brothers, Christine put another tissue just inside his pillowcase, so that Kevin could easily inhale the vapours.

Although initially the smell was quite noticeable, by bedtime it was almost imperceptible. Christine 'recharged' the radiator tissues morning and evening for the following four days, by which time Kevin was definitely much improved. The amazing thing was that not *one* other person in the household caught

Kevin's cold, which totally converted Christine to aromatherapy – she now uses it on all her children, her husband and herself.

Recommended Dosages for All Other Methods of Using Essential Oils

Generally speaking, it is usually safe to use 1 drop of essential oil per 2 stones (12 kg/28 lb) of a child's body weight; for example:

1 – 2 st (6 – 12 kg/14 – 28 lb)	1 drop of essential oil
2 – 4 st (12 – 25 kg/28 – 56 lb)	2 drops
4 – 6 st (25 – 38 kg/56 – 84 lb)	3 drops
6 – 8 st (38 – 50 kg/84 – 112 lb)	4 drops

This dosage is especially important when using baths and other individual treatment methods such as a 'one-off' massage. However, when making up a 50-ml massage oil or lotion to be applied regularly over a long period of time, the general recommended dose for children is 8 drops per 50 ml of carrier oil. This dosage is suitable for all children from the age of one year upwards, because the child's size (i.e. surface area) will determine exactly how much essential oil mixture is used to cover any given part of his body.

However, for children under one year old, use only 5 drops per 50 ml of carrier oil. This is especially important for newborn babies, who have a very active sense of smell and sometimes have very sensitive skin.

Table of Dosages

Weight of child	Number of drops of essential oil in bath, inhalation, compress, etc.	Number of drops of essential oil in 50 ml carrier oil/lotion for massage
Up to 2 st (12 kg/28 lb)	1	5
2 – 4 st (12 – 25 kg/28 – 56 lb)	2	8
4 – 6 st (25 – 38 kg/56 – 84 lb)	3	8
6 – 8 st (38 – 50 kg/84 –112 lb)	4	8
Over 8 st (50 kg/112 lb)	Up to 8	Up to 15

Baths

Bathing with essential oils is a wonderful experience; not only is it relaxing but it can also relieve aches and pains and skin problems too. To use correctly, fill the bath first to the required depth with water (the water should be tepid to warm). The appropriate amount of essential oil drops should then be added using one of the methods below (1 – 3 drops is usually sufficient for a child). Essential oils do not mix easily with water, so it is necessary to swish the water vigorously to disperse the oils. For the most effective treatment the child should remain in the water for 10 full minutes without the addition of bath salts, bubble bath or soap. After the allotted 10 minutes the child can be washed in the normal manner.

As explained in Chapter 3, the essential oils can be added to a carrier before being put into the bath, for example:

- Cream, or the top of the milk; this latter is only useful if you have gold- or silver-top milk. The top of the milk from these is very fatty and the essential oils dissolve fairly well in it. If you then add the cream or milk mixture to the bath water the oils will disperse thoroughly and the cream can give a silky feel to the skin.
- A bland vegetable-based white lotion with no added synthetic perfumes or bleaching agents. Use a dessertspoonful of white lotion and add 1 – 3 drops of essential oils. Shake well and disperse this evenly in the bath by swishing the water thoroughly.

    To make up enough lotion for several baths, add 8 drops of essential oil to 50 ml of lotion and shake well. Use a dessertspoonful of the mixture (15 ml) for each bath (a teaspoonful for a baby), mixing it well with the water. In our opinion this is the best method of using essential oils in a bath for children (or adults!), whether it be a full bath, sitz bath, hand or foot bath.

- Another good way for dispersing your essential oils in the bath is to use honey as the carrier, especially if the child has eczema or psoriasis. (It need not be locally produced honey; the kind you can get at any supermarket is just as good.) One dessertspoonful of runny honey is an excellent carrier for your chosen essential oil. Swish well to disperse the honey (with the essential oils in it) properly throughout the bath.

- A vegetable oil can also be used as a carrier for essential oils in the bath if your child has dry skin. However, care is needed as it may make the bath slippery and unsafe for a child getting in and out if it is not thoroughly dispersed. Nevertheless, if you swish the water really well after adding the drops of essential oils to one teaspoonful of a good carrier like cold-pressed sunflower, for example (or calendula if your child has eczema or psoriasis), there should be no problem.
- If you have access to a pure shampoo base which has no added colouring or synthetic fragrance, then a teaspoonful of this plus your essential oils can be dispersed easily throughout the bath (*see Useful Addresses*). Children enjoy this carrier as it also creates bubbles for them to play with.

Although most essential oils are suitable for the bath, some of the stronger aromas, like lemon, may cause slight skin irritation on a very sensitive child if you exceed the recommended number of drops. Remember that sometimes with aromatherapy, the less you use the better it works.

Adding essential oils to your children's bath is a wonderful idea – not only to help problems from which they may already be suffering, but because using them on a regular basis will help prevent problems occurring in the first place. I [Penny] always add tea tree and lavender to my children's baths as a preventative measure to help keep their immune systems healthy and prevent them from catching the endless rounds of bugs that children seem to pick up at school.

A normal bath is the most useful for skin problems, circulatory problems, aches and pains, hyperactivity and insomnia.

a) Sitz Bath
A sitz bath sounds very grand – in fact a baby bath is fine for this (a washing-up bowl will also do!). In a bath of this size you would still use exactly the same amount of essential oils (1 – 3 drops), but this time always in a carrier, because it is intended to treat the child's bottom, which is often more sensitive than the rest of the body. You would use a sitz bath to treat problems like constipation, intestinal worms, cystitis, thrush, vulval itching, etc.

b) Foot Bath

Again, a baby bath or a washing-up bowl can serve as a foot bath. Add 1 – 3 drops of essential oil, preferably in a carrier, to your tepid water. A foot bath can be used with great effect on the following: athlete's foot, fungal toe nails, sweaty feet, tired or smelly feet, blisters, verrucae and corns.

c) Hand Bath

Your washing-up bowl or a mixing bowl can be used as a hand bath, with 1 – 3 drops of essential oil in a carrier added to the water. Problems that can be helped using a hand bath are dermatitis, fungal fingernails, cuts and bruises, aches and pains. (For the elderly, a hand bath is very effective when treating arthritis in the joints of the fingers.)

Case History

When Ben (aged six) had chicken pox, we made a 50-ml lotion with 3 drops geranium, 2 drops of lemon and 2 drops of Roman chamomile. I asked his mother, Wendy, to put one dessertspoonful of the mixture in Ben's bedtime bath and to apply the lotion directly to the affected areas in the mornings and at lunchtimes.

The bath immediately cooled Ben and relieved the itching caused by the pustules, and his mother felt that, in this particular case, the bath had been the most effective part of the treatment. we asked Wendy to continue with Ben's treatment for seven days to ensure that his recovery was lasting and to help build up his immune system.

Ben's younger brother was also treated with the same mixture and, although he did catch the disease, it was so slight a reaction that Wendy was impressed. She now uses a similar mixture as a matter of course in the boys' baths to help prevent common infections.

Compress

Compresses are a very effective way of using aromatherapy on problems such as bruises, burns, insect bites, sprains, inflammation, etc. Compresses can be either hot or cold. If the problem is on a hand or foot, a sock can be placed over the compress to keep it in place.

1 To make a hot compress, fill a small bowl with hot water – as hot as your hands (and your child) can stand – and add 2 to 3 drops of essential oils, stirring well to disperse them. Make a pad from clean white cotton material (an old handkerchief or tea towel – not medicated lint) and place on the surface of the water to absorb the essential oils. Squeeze lightly and apply the cotton pad to the affected area. To keep the compress in place use ordinary kitchen cling film – this prevents the wetness escaping and also enables the child to move about while the compress is taking effect. Cover with something warm if a hot compress is used.
  A hot compress would be used for muscular aches and pains, bruises, psoriasis, eczema, etc.
2 To make a cold compress, use the above method but use cold water – preferably with ice cubes added.
  A cold compress would be used for insect bites, sprains, inflammation, boils, headaches and swelling.

Large compresses can be kept hot or cold by the application of a hot or cold water-bottle placed on top of the compress. To keep small compresses cold, use a packet of frozen peas or an ice cube twisted in a hanky and put in a plastic bag. For maximum effect the compress should be left in place for at least 30 minutes, although it can be left longer – even overnight, if applied at bedtime. A compress, although simple to apply, is very effective and quickly achieves a good result.

Another method of making a compress is to add your 2 to 3 drops of essential oil to a teaspoonful of carrier lotion or a macerated carrier oil (depending on the problem) and applying it to the affected area. You would then apply your hot or cold cotton to the area and cover as before. This method ensures that the essential oils go directly to the heart of the problem.

Case History

When Alison's horse stood on her foot, her mother, a trainee aromatherapist, phoned us for advice. Alison was 13 years old at the time. After discussion, we decided to use 2 drops of cypress, 1 drop of lavender and 1 drop of rosemary in a teaspoonful of hypericum (St John's wort) oil, to help against bruising and to relieve the pain.

Half of this mixture was applied to Alison's foot and lower leg, which was then wrapped in a cotton compress and plastic film, then covered with a crepe bandage. We did not use any extremes of temperature. The compress was left on for one hour while Alison was lying down. The remaining mixture was then applied in small doses twice more at hourly intervals.

In this short space of time Alison's foot was nearly as good as new, with very little swelling or bruising. After two days and two further compresses, there was absolutely no sign of her injury.

Alison herself was so pleased with the result that she used the same oils and treatment method when her horse Trigger bruised his own leg – and had equally good results!

Neat Application

Usually essential oils are not applied neat to the skin. However, there are certain emergency situations where essential oils can be applied neat to great effect, for example insect bites, cuts, burns and wounds. Usually only oils like tea tree, *Eucalyptus smithii*, lavender and geranium are applied neat to the skin, and this should only be done as a 'one off' treatment followed up with another method of application when the emergency is over.

Case Histories

When Victor was only nine months old his foot was accidentally trapped in the car door. Immediately Penny applied 4 drops of lavender directly onto the already swollen area, which was beginning to show signs of bruising.

She then took Victor to the local casualty department to check for any damage. By the time we were seen by a nurse (30 minutes later) there was hardly any evidence of injury – in fact she had to ask which foot had been damaged!

Fortunately, the X-ray showed no broken bones (incidentally, he had to be wakened for the X-ray, so presumably by then he was in no great pain!). The next morning there was still no obvious difference at all between his feet, no bruising and no swelling.

Edward was rather prone to cold sores but never actually suffers any more due to prompt treatment with neat *Eucalyptus smithii*. As soon as he felt the 'tingling' sensation of a cold sore, he applied neat *E. smithii* directly onto the area. After just one day of several applications, the tingling died down and the cold sore never actually appeared.

Massage

Instead of mixing 1 or 2 drops of essential oil in a carrier every time your child wants a massage, it is much more practical to make up 50 ml of massage oil at a time. The recommended dose is 8 drops of essential oil to every 50 ml of carrier oil (*see page 65*). Eight drops in 50 ml gives the right amount of drops per ml of carrier for the two year old up to the 12 year old (*see page 65 for babies under two*). This is because for a two–year–old far less carrier oil or lotion will be used than for a 12–year–old, as obviously the surface area of the child's skin is going to limit the amount you can apply in any one treatment.

NB When using three or four essential oils in a treatment it is a good idea to put them together in one dropper bottle (as recommended on *page 66*). With this method you can make massage oils or lotions easily and economically and have a neat essential oil mixture to use for the bath, to inhale or to use in the next bottle of carrier oil or lotion.

Massage is useful for enhancing a child/parent bond, for relaxation, insomnia, stress, aches and pains, sluggish circulation, as a digestive tonic and also as a means of passive exercise for your child (*see Chapter 6*). It is not always necessary to complete a whole body massage on your child. He can benefit from small parts of his body being massaged, for example the abdomen when he has colic, or the legs after a sports day at school, etc. A back massage at bedtime is extremely beneficial, enabling your child to relax, to feel comforted, warmed and ready for sleep. (*See Chapter 6 for massage techniques.*)

NB After making up your 50 ml of massage oil it must be labelled – and stored in a dark glass bottle with the lid tightly screwed on to prevent rancidity. Also, keep it in a dark place such as a cupboard, as light damages essential oils and encourages rancidity. Glass bottles are preferable to plastic, as essential oils can attack certain brittle types of plastic.

Case Histories

Debbie, an aromatherapist, treats a little boy with cerebral palsy who comes to her on a weekly basis (he has a twin brother who is a healthy and sprightly child). Lawrence is very big for his six years and very strong. He has been coming for massage now for almost three years and was quite a tot when he first began treatment. He is very energetic and on the go all the time. He is also quite vocal, and treatments involve a lot of shouting and squealing.

Debbie uses lavender, sandalwood and Roman chamomile to massage his legs, arms, chest (he is prone to coughs) and back. His mother and Debbie sometimes wonder whether he actually relaxes at all, though he does imitate the movements on himself and occasionally his eyes close while Debbie is working on certain areas.

His mum thinks he has benefited overall and his muscle tone is fantastic for a child his age, which she thinks suits him, hence his physical strength. She jokes that we will have to tie him down one day, as she is sure he will eventually bounce right off the couch during his treatment!

Debbie's daughter Emily's favourite essential oil is Roman chamomile – her mother believes this is due to her influence as she used it a lot during her pregnancy, together with lavender and frankincense in a carrier oil, to rub onto her tummy to help prevent stretch marks. Once Debbie applied the same oils to her buttocks when she was in agony with sciatica and the pain went away within 10 minutes.

Debbie makes a diluted blend of Roman chamomile in sweet almond oil to massage Emily's tummy and back. This helps to relax her at night if she is over-excited. She especially likes her shoulders and back massaged, as she is then 'like nana' (Debbie gives her own mum a regular neck and shoulder massage).

Hair Treatments

- Shampoo – add 8 drops of essential oil or chosen essential oils to 50 ml of good quality base shampoo *containing no synthetic perfumes or colourings.* Use a teaspoonful each time you wash your child's hair. This method of treatment can be used to treat dandruff, greasy hair, dry hair, fine hair, psoriasis and lice, depending on your choice of oils.

- Hair rinse – put 8 drops of essential oil into a narrow-necked bottle containing 50 ml of water. After the hair has been shampooed and towel dried as normal, apply to and spread along the scalp, repeating till the whole scalp is covered, then combing to the ends of the hair. This treatment is very beneficial in the treatment of lice and nits (*see below*).

Regarding certain plant extracts affecting the colour of the hair, as explained in Chapter 1, distillation only extracts the smallest (and volatile) molecules from a plant. Different methods of extraction enable other, larger molecules to be extracted and it is these which are used to effect a colour change on the hair. For example, chamomile extract is said to lighten blonde hair; an extract from the ripe green outer shell of the walnut will enhance the colour of brown hair, etc.

Essential oils can be used as follows, to add a little lustre and also an aroma to the hair. Lemon and Roman chamomile add shine to blonde hair, and ylang ylang, geranium and sandalwood add lustre to brunettes.

However, there are essential oils which will assist dry hair, greasy hair, and lifeless or thin hair – and also hair which is falling out (*see Chapter 2*).

- Scalp tonic – add 8 drops of your chosen essential oil to 50 ml of pure distilled water and keep the mixture in a dark brown bottle. Make partings in the hair and apply a little of the scalp tonic directly to your child's scalp itself, rather than the hair, then distribute it evenly over the scalp with your fingertips. Massage his head as follows immediately after applying the tonic: place your fingers firmly on your child's scalp and move the skin over the skull underneath (that is, don't just move your fingers through his hair). This improves circulation, which in turn will encourage healthy hair growth. Scalp tonic is useful for dry, brittle hair or where the hair growth is feeble, thin, fine or impaired. The tonic can be left to dry into the hair.

- Scalp oil – add 8 drops of your chosen essential oil to 50 ml of carrier oil and keep in a dark brown bottle. Apply as for scalp tonic, creating partings throughout the hair and applying the oil directly onto the scalp. Scalp oil can be used to treat cradle cap, dandruff, psoriasis, eczema and dry skin, also insect bites and lice which may be on the scalp itself. Leave the oil on the hair for at least one hour before shampooing with a good quality shampoo and following with a hair rinse (*see above*).

NB For the common problem of lice and nits, essential oils of rosemary, *Eucalyptus smithii* and sweet thyme are most successful, avoiding the use of chemicals which may harm your child's skin and hair. The regular use of an essential oil hair rinse will deter nits and lice and can be used as a very effective preventative.

When using water-based mixtures like the scalp tonic and the hair rinse, make sure that you always shake the bottle well before application to ensure thorough dispersion of the essential oil throughout the water.

Case Histories

When Toby (six) came home with head lice, Penny immediately made up a shampoo containing rosemary, *E. smithii* and sweet thyme. She applied this to his dry hair and covered his head with a swimming cap for 10 minutes. After rinsing thoroughly, she applied a hair rinse using one cupful (300 ml) of water with 2 drops each of the same oils, following this by combing his hair with a fine-toothed comb. The result was instant and, because Toby has asthma, she was pleased to note that the treatment had not affected his breathing, as can sometimes happen with a proprietary brand treatment.

After treating the rest of the household, Penny ensured that the problem did not recur by using the shampoo once a week.

When five-year-old Sarah's parents decided to separate, apart from being withdrawn, her hair began to fall out in large handfuls.

We recommended a scalp tonic using rosemary, ylang ylang and rosewood in equal proportions (to help stimulate the circulation and reduce stress). The tonic was to be applied twice a day to the scalp immediately prior to a five-minute scalp massage (*see Chapter 6*). Initially Sarah's hair seemed to fall out even more. We reassured her mother that this was normal, as the loosened hairs were being shed more quickly. However, in just one week Sarah's hair loss had slowed down. By the end of the third week of this daily treatment, hair loss had become minimal, and Sarah's hair was looking much healthier and glossier.

We also suggested that Sarah should use the same three oils in the bath. We mixed 10 drops of each oil in a small bottle with a dropper insert and recommended that her mother disperse 2 – 3 drops thoroughly in Sarah's evening bath to help reduce the stress she was obviously going through.

With prolonged use (and her lovely mother's attentive care!) Sarah began to sleep more at night and appeared much less withdrawn during the day. She is now seven, and will not have a bath without 'her' oils.

Mouth Wash

Add 4 drops of your chosen essential oils to 50 ml of distilled water and keep in a brown glass bottle. Each time, before using, make sure you agitate the bottle thoroughly to ensure dispersion of the essential oils throughout the water. Pour a small amount of the mouth wash into a clean glass and ask your child to take a mouthful and swish the mixture around in his mouth for 30 seconds. He could also gargle with the mixture before spitting it down the sink. If you are unsure whether your child can gargle effectively, try with plain water first. Ask your child not to swallow the mouth wash; however, accidentally swallowing a small amount will not harm him. Mouth washes can be used effectively to fight gum disease, thrush, mouth ulcers, bad breath, abscesses, toothache and sore throats.

Case History

Kylie (seven) was suffering from mouth ulcers. We mixed up a mouth wash using 5 drops of bergamot and 3 drops sweet orange in 100 ml distilled water. Kylie was asked to stir the mixture well and gargle thoroughly, swishing the water around in her mouth before spitting it out.

She did this three times during the first day and was pleased to tell us that the pain had gone from the ulcers. We asked her not to eat too much sugary food and to continue the treatment for one further day, by which time the ulcers had subsided.

Now, whenever Kylie feels the ulcers returning she asks for a mouth wash. These times are getting very few and far between now and, in conjunction with a healthy diet, Kylie rarely has a recurrence of the problem.

Oils/Lotions/Creams

For massage, a carrier oil is a better medium than lotion as it takes longer to be absorbed into your child's skin, thus enabling an easy flowing massage to take place and creating a silky feel to the skin.

However, if you just wish to apply essential oils in a carrier to an affected area, a bland lotion or cream is more comfortable for a child than using a vegetable oil. Constant use of a carrier oil can stain clothing and make the child's skin feel greasy or sticky – this does not happen when using a lotion or cream.

Always ensure that your creams and lotions are pure and natural (vegetable based) and do not contain any mineral oil, synthetic perfumes, colours or preservatives. To every 50 ml of vegetable oil, lotion or cream add 8 drops of the essential oils of your choice (5 if the child is under two). Skin lotions and creams are useful in cases of psoriasis, eczema, dermatitis, poor circulation, localized pain, etc.

Case Histories

Emily suffers with colds which always lead to chesty coughs. Night-times are the worst as she seems to get more congested.

Her mother, Debbie, who is an aromatherapist, found that 3 or 4 drops of *Eucalyptus smithii* on a tissue in the pillow slip and a chest rub of *E. smithii*, sweet marjoram and cedarwood mixed in a lotion and applied at bedtime helped to dry out the congestion and also helped Emily to sleep well.

Janine, a very pretty nine-year-old, loves swimming. Unfortunately, because of her eczema she used to be unable to swim often as the chlorine exacerbated the problem. The eczema was behind her ears, elbows and knees, and at times became so painful and itchy that Janine was reduced to tears.

After talking to Margaret, her mother, it was discovered that Janine's father and paternal grandmother also had eczema. We discussed Janine's diet in great detail and found that she had a large amount of dairy produce in her diet. Margaret agreed to eliminate cheese and cow's milk from Janine's diet and to increase her intake of fresh green vegetables and fruit.

We mixed up 50 ml of calendula and sunflower oils with essential oils of bergamot, geranium and lavender – to be applied to the affected areas twice daily and before swimming.

After just two weeks the eczema had stopped weeping and was beginning to heal. Margaret was told that she could reduce the applications to once a day (and before swimming) to control the eczema.

Now, Janine has almost no evidence of eczema, except at times of stress (swimming galas!) when Margaret takes extra care to apply the oil.

As a 'side-effect', Janine's sinuses became clearer – a result I believe of her improved diet – and she can now swim with no discomfort.

Harry and his son Jonathan (11) both had athlete's foot. They told us they were keen squash players and because of this (so they thought) they both suffered from sweaty feet.

We assured them that athletes should not have to endure sweaty feet or athlete's foot more than any other member of society, especially if care is taken with footwear. After discussing the virtues of pure cotton socks, cotton pumps and leather trainers/shoes, we asked them both to show us their feet!

Father and son had damp, cool feet and the athlete's foot fungus (*tinea pedis*) was evident between the toes, where it had caused severe splitting of the skin.

We already have a good base cream in a 50-ml pot (called, incidentally, Calming Moisture Cream, which is especially formulated for skin conditions [*see Useful Addresses*]) and we added 3 drops tea tree, 3 drops geranium and 2 drops of lavender to this base cream, asking Harry and Jonathan to use it three times daily. We also asked them, when possible, to go barefoot after applying the cream, to allow the air to circulate and help prevent the infection spreading. They assured us they would do this, and that they would wear 100 per cent cotton socks. We also asked them to cut down on sugary, yeasty foods until their condition improved.

We did not see either of them for a month. When we did, Jonathan's athlete's foot had cleared up totally. Harry's was still evident, however, so we mixed him some more cream to last another month. Towards the end of the second month we had a phone call from Harry for more cream. We were rather worried that his feet were taking so long to clear, and enquired about this. He told me that the cream was not for him at all, because his problem had cleared up, but for another chap at the squash club who had athlete's foot!

Bathing Wounds

Add 4 drops of essential oil to 50 ml of warm clean boiled water and wipe down the wound or the cut as necessary, using oils that are highly antiseptic yet non-irritating, like tea tree and *Eucalyptus smithii*. This method of treatment is also a useful follow-up after using neat essential oil on an insect bite, as it is cooling to the area. Never bathe the eyes with essential oils, even if diluted in water or a carrier oil. Always buy a proprietary brand of eye drops (such as Chamomile Eye Care – *see Useful Addresses and below*).

Case History

Penny was due to teach an advanced aromatherapy course in Israel in the summer of 1994 and had decided to take the opportunity to extend her visit (together with the family) to have a holiday. She forgot to pack her usual oils (lavender, tea tree and *Eucalyptus smithii*) to be used in emergency situations.

Fortunately, the course organizer asked her to bring a dozen bottles of chamomile hydrolat as it was very popular with her clients. She duly packed the hydrolats, taking an extra six bottles in case any of the students were interested in trying them.

She will always be grateful that she did! For Penny it became a 'rescue remedy' for her children – she used it for everything! Just to name a few of the conditions successfully treated: sunburn, cuts, bruises, diarrhoea, tummy ache, headache, insect bites and skin rashes.

Plasters/Bandages

Most children, when they have a cut or wound, like to wear a plaster or bandage to display it proudly to their friends. Don't disappoint them; simply put 1 drop of neat essential oil such as tea tree, lavender or *Eucalyptus smithii* on the lint part of the plaster and apply as normal. This will ensure speedy healing while having an antiseptic effect on the wound. If applying a bandage use 1 or 2 drops of essential oil on a piece of damp lint, apply to the wound and bandage as normal.

Conclusion

As you can see, there are many methods of application in different carriers for essential oils. One condition may call for only one method, another several; also, some people prefer certain methods of use over others. This is fine. The main criteria is that when your child is happy with both the smell and the chosen method, it is then right for him. Provided that the percentage of essential oil to carrier does not exceed the recommended dose, you can be assured of a totally safe, natural method of helping Mother Nature to do her job.

Household Hints

There are many ways of using essential oils for environmental fragrancing, for instance in daily tasks around the home, just to make the atmosphere around you more pleasant.

- Neat essential oil will remove oil-based marker-pen stains from your children's hands.
- If planning a children's party, use 4 – 8 drops of an appropriate oil (such as one of the citrus oils) in a vaporizer. For a mixed-ages party, rosemary and lavender together are ideal. For a dinner party for two, something exotic like ylang ylang is always pleasant.
- Putting 3 – 4 drops of tea tree in the toilet bowl kills all bacteria and germs completely and is also environmentally friendly.
- To remove chewing gum from fabric or hair, first cover the area with ice cubes covered in plastic. When really cold, pick off as much surplus gum as possible. Then, using a soft clean cloth with neat *Eucalyptus smithii*, hold over the area for one minute. The gum will dissolve away.

- By filling the ashtray in your car with *unscented* pot pourri (*see Useful Addresses*) and then fragrancing it with essential oils you can create a healthy and pleasant environment within the car. It is especially useful if you or your children suffer from travel sickness – you can use the appropriate essential oils for this particular problem. (If you add rosemary and lemon to your pot pourri mixture it will help to keep you awake while driving long distances.)
- To remove sticky label marks, use a few drops of almost any essential oil on a piece of cloth.
- Add 2 – 3 drops of essential oils to the water compartment of your steam iron – ironing will never be as boring again with the wonderful smell of essential oils coming to you as you perform this tedious task.
  Caution: If the water well of your iron is made of brittle plastic, it may craze.
- Putting 6 – 8 drops of essential oil on a cotton wool ball placed in your vacuum cleaner bag can fragrance the room as you clean, creating a pleasant smell.
- Adding essential oils to *unscented* pot pourri can also make the environment congenial and friendly.
- Essential oils, as they are antiseptic, can be used to wipe down work surfaces. Many of them are also antiviral. Add 4 – 5 drops to 1 pint (600 ml) of warm water and wipe down surfaces as normal. Not only does this create a pleasant smell but it also kills germs and is environmentally friendly.
- Put 5 – 6 drops of your favourite oil in the final rinse of your wash cycle. Then if you have to dry clothes indoors, at least you can enjoy the fresh smell.
- When airing the beds, use 4 – 5 drops of oil to 1 pint (600 ml) of water in a spray bottle. Spray lightly over the bed and allow to dry naturally before remaking the beds. This not only fragrances the room but also helps prevent bed bugs, dust mites and airborne infection.

- **Try seasonal fragrancing**:
  - For Christmas, put drops of frankincense, rosewood and orange on pine cones. Put these near a warm place or burn them in an open fire.
  - In January, vaporize sandalwood and rosemary to keep the blues at bay. A lovely spring-time mixture can be made from sweet marjoram, Roman chamomile and lavender.

- Summertime smells would include rose otto, geranium and sweet thyme. For crisp autumn days try cedarwood, cypress and ginger, which make a truly warming, woody mixture.
- For dark, damp, muggy weather, lighten the atmosphere with *Eucalyptus smithii*, bergamot and mandarin.

Cookery Tips

When using essential oils in cooking, always drop the oils onto a teaspoon first to prevent overflavouring the food.

1 Add 5 – 6 drops of lemon or orange oil to a basic Victoria sponge (cake) recipe.
2 Add 4 drops of ginger to a standard biscuit recipe for extra flavour.
3 Christmas cakes and puddings always benefit from 4 – 5 drops of ginger and lemon essential oils.
4 For perfect roast lamb, put 1 drop of rosemary in a dessertspoonful of warm honey and brush over the joint. Cook for the first hour covered in tin foil, then as normal.
5 To flavour bottled water, to every litre add 3 drops of lemon, mandarin or orange essential oils. Shake well before serving with slices of fruit.

5

Common Ailments A – Z

Precautions

Please remember that aromatherapy is not to be used in place of medical care. Contact your doctor at once if your child has any of the following symptoms:

- A temperature of 39°C (102°F) or over
- Cannot be woken
- Has a fit or convulsion
- Is unusually 'floppy'
- Refuses two feeds in succession
- Seems to be in severe pain
- Has inhaled a foreign body into the lungs
- Passes stools that are red or white
- Has persistent sickness and diarrhoea
- Has breathing difficulties, or has turned blue
- Has an obvious infection or illness
- Has signs of meningitis (headache, stiff neck, high temperature, sensitive eyes)

If you think your child is in danger, phone the emergency services (999 in the UK; 911 in the US) and ask for urgent assistance.

Always listen to your own maternal or paternal instincts where the health of your child is concerned – you are usually right!

Remember that prevention is always easier and better than having to cure – and this is where your aromatherapy oils can be invaluable. Regular use of the correct essential oils used in a vaporizer, bath or massage will help to keep your children free from many of the problems that can affect them – particularly when they start school.

Caring for Your Sick Child

Remember that alongside medical and/or aromatherapy treatment you can help your child's discomfort by being aware of the following:

1 Keep your child comfortably cool. Do not be tempted to wrap up a sick child to keep him warm, as the body temperature will usually rise naturally to help fight infection. Keeping your child too warm will increase his feelings of illness. Use light coverings and, if necessary, sponge him down with tepid water containing 2 – 3 drops *Eucalyptus smithii.*
2 Give plenty of fluids. Water is obviously the best fluid to give your child as it will flush the body of toxins and improve the functions of the excretory organs, enabling them to rid the body of toxins quickly. Fluids also prevent dehydration. If your child does not like water, try it in the form of ice cubes or flavour the water (as described on *page 69*) with a few drops of essential oils.
3 Let your child eat what he fancies (within reason), as his body will dictate to a certain extent whatever is needed.
4 Let your child stay close to you. Bed rest is just as effective on the sofa! Perhaps a soothing massage would also be beneficial at this time, keeping well covered the parts of the body not being massaged.

Common Problems

Some of the following sections include a sample recipe, but please refer to Chapter 4 for dosages and methods of use and see also Chapter 7 for a full range of health queries your child may develop.

Abdominal Pain

All children get tummy ache from time to time, from colic in young babies to indigestion in an older child. If your child is older, ask him to explain where the pain is and how it feels. A young baby will draw up his knees if in pain and cry. This is usually wind (in our experience), but if you are worried call the doctor.

Treatment
- Babies and children: If breastfeeding, the mother can drink fennel or chamomile tea; the therapeutic properties will be passed directly to the baby via the mother's milk.
- Bath
- Massage
- Compress
- Recommended carriers: calendula, sunflower, white lotion
- Recommended essential oils: chamomile (Roman), ginger, lavender, mandarin, marjoram (sweet), sandalwood

Suggested Recipes
- Bath:
    1 drop chamomile (Roman) (*Chamaemelum nobile*)
    1 drop mandarin (*Citrus reticulata*)
- Massage oil:
    10 ml calendula oil
    40 ml sunflower oil
    3 drops ginger (*Zingiber officinale*)
    3 drops lavender (*Lavandula angustifolia*)
    2 drops chamomile (Roman) (*Chamaemelum nobile*)
    Label the bottle for future use
- Compress:
    1 tsp white lotion
    1 man-sized hanky
    1 drop ginger (*Zingiber officinale*)
    1 drop lavender (*Lavandula angustifolia*)
    1 drop sandalwood (*Santalum album*)
    Apply half the mixture over the abdomen – *see page 69* for full method (may be useful on children)

Allergies

An allergy is an abnormal response of the body's immune system to an 'allergen' or 'irritant'. Allergies tend to run in families. Common irritants include household dust, pollen, chemicals, perfume, animal hair and certain foods. (*See also* **Asthma**, **Eczema** and **Hayfever**)

Treatment
- Bath
- Massage
- Face and body lotion
- Recommended carriers: calendula, cream, grapeseed, sunflower, white lotion
- Recommended essential oils: bergamot*, chamomile (Roman), geranium*, lavender*

Suggested Recipes
- Bath:
    1 drop geranium (*Pelargonium graveolens*)
    1 drop lavender (*Lavandula angustifolia*)
- Massage oil:
    10 ml calendula oil
    10 ml sunflower oil
    30 ml grapeseed oil
    3 drops geranium (*Pelargonium graveolens*)
    2 drops chamomile (Roman) (*Chamaemelum nobile*)
    2 drops lavender (*Lavandula angustifolia*)
    1 drop bergamot (*Citrus bergamia*)
- Face and body lotion:
    50 ml bland white lotion
    4 drops lavender (*Lavandula angustifolia*)
    3 drops bergamot (*Citrus bergamia*)
    3 drops geranium (*Pelargonium graveolens*)

Anxiety

Probably anxiety is suffered more by children than adults realize! Changing school routines, starting nursery, being unwell, being affected by parents' squabbles or even separation, or simply being over-stimulated by well-meaning but over-exacting parents can all lead to a stressful child. Symptoms can include a worsening of allergies (such as asthma), sleeplessness, loss of appetite, constipation or diarrhoea and a pallid skin – among many others.

Treatment
- Bath
- Massage
- Vaporization
- Inhalation (for panic attacks)
- Recommended carriers: avocado, hypericum, lime blossom, sunflower
- Recommended essential oils: bergamot, chamomile (Roman), geranium, lavender, mandarin, marjoram (sweet), orange (sweet), rose otto, rosewood*, sandalwood*, thyme (sweet), ylang ylang

Suggested Recipes
- Vaporization:
    2 drops rosewood (*Aniba rosaeodora*)
    2 drops ylang ylang (*Cananga odorata*)
- Massage oil:
    30 ml lime blossom
    20 ml sunflower oil
    3 drops geranium (*Pelargonium graveolens*)
    3 drops sandalwood (*Santalum album*)
    2 drops ylang ylang (*Cananga odorata*)

Asthma

Asthma is caused by a narrowing of the bronchial tubes, usually in response to an allergen. It tends to run in families and can also be brought on by exercise or by inhaling smoke, perfume or petrol fumes. Usually the sufferer has a frequent cough, wheezing, breathlessness or colds which do not seem to clear. It is thought that 1 in 10 children has asthma in varying degrees and that it is more common in boys than girls. An asthma attack can be extremely frightening for a child, so treatment must always be undertaken in association with your GP.

Treatment
- Vaporization (without steam)
- Face lotion (*see* **Allergies**)
- Chest massage
- Recommended carriers: sunflower, white lotion
- Recommended essential oils: *Eucalyptus smithii*, frankincense, lavender, mandarin, marjoram (sweet), rose otto, thyme (sweet)

Suggested Recipe
- Massage oil:
    - 50 ml sunflower oil
    - 3 drops lavender (*Lavandula angustifolia*)
    - 3 drops thyme (sweet) (*Thymus vulgaris* linalool or geraniol chemotype)
    - 2 drops mandarin (*Citrus reticulata*)

Athlete's Foot

This is a fungal infection of the skin on the feet. Usually found between the toes, the skin can be painful, itchy and cracked; often a cheesy smell accompanies the condition.

Treatment
- Foot bath
- Foot lotion
- Recommended carriers: calendula, grapeseed, white lotion or cream
- Recommended essential oils: geranium, lavender, tea tree

Suggested Recipes
- Foot bath:
    - 1 drop geranium (*Pelargonium graveolens*)
    - 1 drop tea tree (*Melaleuca alternifolia*)
- Foot lotion:
    - 50 ml white lotion
    - 3 drops lavender (*Lavandula angustifolia*)
    - 3 drops tea tree (*Melaleuca alternifolia*)
    - 2 drops geranium (*Pelargonium graveolens*)

Bedwetting

This can be very distressing for a child (*see* **Anxiety**) and also for you, the parent. There are several causes, ranging from an incompetent bladder sphincter muscle, to stress, or an inability to wake from deep sleep. The best approach is to remain calm and never chastise a child for his 'accidents'. Eventually he should grow out of this, although to help him you could 'lift' him before you go to bed, so that his bladder is emptied at least once in the proper place during the night. In our experience this is not a cure, however – since the child has not had to learn to do this for himself – but it can at least save unnecessary washing of bedlinen. Restricting drinks before bedtime can also help.

Treatment
- Bath
- Abdomen massage (lower back before bed)
- Recommended carriers: hypericum
- Recommended essential oils: cypress, marjoram (sweet)*, rosemary

NB Bottled or cooled boiled water is best for your child. Tea, coffee, cola drinks and hot chocolate are not good for children because they are not only stimulants but also diuretics, which could place unnecessary further stress on a child's bladder.

Suggested Recipe
- Bath:
     2 drops cypress (*Cupressus sempervirens*)
     1 drop marjoram (sweet) (*Origanum majorana*)

Blisters

Blisters can be caused by the continual rubbing of two surfaces together, for example new shoes can cause blisters on the heel or tops of the toes, and too much writing done by a child just learning to write can cause blisters on the fingers.

Treatment
- Compress
- Lotion application
- Recommended carriers: calendula, hypericum, rose hip, sunflower, white lotion

- Recommended essential oils: cedarwood, cypress, geranium, lavender, orange (sweet)

Suggested Recipe
- Compress:
    2 drops cypress (*Cupressus sempervirens*)
    1 drop geranium (*Pelargonium graveolens*)
    1 drop lavender (*Lavandula angustifolia*)

Bronchitis

This is caused by inflammation of the bronchi (air passages) and usually progresses from a simple cold, runny nose and raised temperature. The child will cough and produce phlegm – which can be painful, more so at night.

Check with your doctor that your child has bronchitis and not bronchiolitis, which is a viral infection (or which can be a form of asthma).

Treatment
- Bath
- Chest massage
- Vaporization
- Recommended carriers: hypericum, sunflower, white lotion
- Recommended essential oils: cedarwood, cypress, *Eucalyptus smithii*, frankincense, lavender, marjoram (sweet), rosemary, rose otto, rosewood, sandalwood, tea tree, thyme (sweet)

Suggested Recipe
- Massage oil:
    10 ml hypericum (St John's wort)
    40 ml sunflower oil
    3 drops cedarwood (*Cedrus atlantica*)
    3 drops thyme (sweet) (*Thymus vulgaris* linalool or geraniol chemotype)
    2 drops tea tree (*Melaleuca alternifolia*)

Bruises

Bruises occur usually after a sharp knock on a part of the body, or after falling over, etc. The blood capillaries in the area are temporarily damaged and blood floods the affected area, causing discolouration.

Treatment
- Compress
- Lotion application
- Recommended carriers: calendula, hypericum, olive, rose hip, white lotion
- Recommended essential oils: cypress, *Eucalyptus smithii*, lavender*, lemon*, rosemary

Suggested Recipe
- Lotion:
    10 ml hypericum (St John's wort)
    10 ml rose hip
    30 ml white lotion
    4 drops cypress (*Cupressus sempervirens*)
    2 drops *Eucalyptus smithii*
    2 drops rosemary (*Rosmarinus officinalis*)

Burns (minor)

Minor burns can be treated very successfully with aromatherapy. First ensure that the burn has been doused with cold water for at least five minutes or until the extreme heat has gone out of it.

Treatment
- Initial application of neat lavender followed by one of the carrier oils below, or white lotion containing essential oils.
- Recommended carriers: carrot, hypericum, olive, rose hip, white lotion
- Recommended essential oils: chamomile (Roman), frankincense, lavender, rosemary, rose otto

Suggested Recipe
- Lotion application:
    50 ml white lotion
    4 drops lavender (*Lavandula angustifolia*)
    2 drops frankincense (*Boswellia carteri*)
    2 drops rose otto (*Rosa damascena*)

Chicken Pox

The chicken pox virus is incubated for 12 to 20 days before symptoms appear.
The child then develops a temperature, feels unwell – and small, red, itchy
spots begin to erupt over the chest, trunk and eventually the face. These
spots blister and eventually form crusts.

Treatment
- Baths
- Application (on affected areas)
- Adding a tea-cup full of bicarbonate of soda (as well as essential oils) to the
  bath water is beneficial.
- Recommended carriers: carrot oil, white lotion
- Recommended essential oils: chamomile (Roman), frankincense, geranium,
  lavender, lemon*, rose otto

Suggested Recipe
- Application lotion:
    20 ml carrot oil
    30 ml white lotion
    3 drops geranium (*Pelargonium graveolens*)
    3 drops lavender (*Lavandula angustifolia*)
    2 drops lemon (*Citrus limon*)

Chilblains

These are common in children in the winter and are due to poor circulation.
They are painful purplish red swellings on the toes and fingers that can be very
inflamed and itchy.

Treatment
- Foot bath/hand bath
- Foot/hand lotion
- Recommended carriers: calendula, carrot, sunflower, sweet almond, white lotion
- Recommended essential oils: chamomile (Roman), cypress, lavender, lemon, sandalwood*

Suggested Recipes
- Foot bath:
    1 drop lemon (*Citrus limon*)
    1 drop sandalwood (*Santalum album*)
- Application lotion:
    50 ml white lotion
    2 drops chamomile (Roman) (*Chamaemelum nobile*)
    2 drops lavender (*Lavandula angustifolia*)
    2 drops lemon (*Citrus limon*)
    2 drops sandalwood (*Santalum album*)

Cold Sores

Cold sores are caused by the herpes simplex virus, which remains dormant for long periods in the tri-geminal facial nerve (at the temples). From time to time the virus flares up, producing small groups of blisters which fill up with yellow fluid and feel hot and itchy. Cold sores can be triggered by stress, sunshine, wind or cold weather, or the common cold. Ice cubes applied to the area can help to relieve the pain. A person with herpes should avoid contact with other people, especially children with eczema, as this can trigger an infection.[1] Once a child has contracted the virus, the cold sore can reappear in the identical spot whenever his health is at a low ebb, such as if he is suffering from a cold or is stressed.

Treatment
- Direct application to lip and also to temples (where the herpes virus lies dormant between attacks)
- Lotion
- Bath
- Recommended carriers: hypericum (St John's Wort), white lotion
- Recommended essential oils: *Eucalyptus smithii*, geranium, lavender

Suggested Recipe
- Application of any one of the essential oils listed above directly on to the cold sore with a cotton bud (dipped first in hypericum oil) every 2 hours for the first day. After this the application lotion or hypericum should be used, except for one direct application per day, preferably just before bedtime.
- Application lotion:
    - 1 tsp white lotion
    - 2 drops *Eucalyptus smithii*
    - 1 drop geranium (*Pelargonium graveolens*)
    - 1 drop lavender (*Lavandula angustifolia*)

Colic

Most babies in the first few months of life are at times said to be suffering from colic. With this the baby cries shrilly (usually for a period in the evening) and draws up his knees as if in pain (*see* **Abdominal Pain**). It is presumed that bubbles of air have become trapped in the baby's intestines, causing pain. Sometimes the abdomen can become distended.

Treatment
- Tea
- Bath
- Massage
- Recommended carriers: calendula, grapeseed, white lotion
- Recommended essential oils: bergamot, chamomile (Roman), ginger, lavender, mandarin, marjoram (sweet), rosemary, ylang ylang

Suggested Recipe
- If breastfeeding, the mother can drink chamomile or fennel tea, or ginger beer during the day: this will then be conveyed to the baby via the breastmilk.
- Very weak chamomile tea (very weak chamomile drink, given in small amounts late in the afternoon prior to feeding) can be helpful.
- Massage oil:
    - 10 ml calendula oil
    - 40 ml grapeseed oil
    - 3 drops ginger (*Zingiber officinale*)
    - 3 drops mandarin (*Citrus reticulata*)
    - 2 drops chamomile (Roman) (*Chamaemelum nobile*)

Common Cold

Colds are caused by many different types of cold viruses. Often young children seem to have one long continual cold, while in fact it may be one viral attack after another. As children grow, colds become less frequent as they become immune to the several differing viruses.

Treatment
- Bath
- Vaporization
- Neck and chest rubs
- Recommended carriers: carrot (for inflammation), grapeseed, sunflower, white lotion
- Recommended essential oils: cedarwood, *Eucalyptus smithii*, lemon, rosemary, rose otto, sandalwood*, tea tree, thyme (sweet)

Suggested Recipe
- Chest rub:
    20 ml hypericum (St John's wort)
    30 ml sunflower oil
    4 drops tea tree (*Melaleuca alternifolia*)
    2 drops lemon (*Citrus limon*)
    2 drops rose otto (*Rosa damascena*)

Conjunctivitis

This is usually caused by a bacterial or viral infection but may also be triggered by a foreign body in the eye. The eyes become painful, red and watery and sometimes produce pus as a result of the delicate membrane covering the white of the eye becoming inflamed. Sometimes called 'pink eye'.

Treatment
- Bathe eyes with cooled boiled water, using separate pieces of cotton wool for each eye.
- DO NOT USE ESSENTIAL OILS.

Constipation

This happens when the bowels are not opened regularly (every one to two days) and the faeces become compacted, hard and dry. Sometimes emotional upset or a poor diet can bring on constipation too. It could also happen if the child is rushed or hurried and simply not given enough time to open his bowels in a relaxed manner. Start training as early as is viable for you and your baby; notice what time of day your baby is opening his bowels (in his nappy) and put him on his potty after the meal which is nearest to, and before, the movement. Praise him each time he is successful and gradually he will acquire the habit of going regularly at that time of day.

Treatment
• Bath
• Abdomen massage
• Encourage your child to take time on the toilet, and to drink plenty of cool boiled water. Make sure he is comfortable on his potty or trainer seat and try to give him a diet high in fruits and vegetables. The best preventative solution is to encourage him to 'try' at the same time each day – after breakfast is an ideal time. Once in operation, this can then develop into a habit.
• Recommended carriers: avocado, sunflower
• Recommended essential oils: ginger, mandarin, orange (sweet), rosemary

Suggested Recipe
• Abdomen massage oil:
    20 ml avocado oil
    30 ml sunflower oil
    3 drops ginger (*Zingiber officinale*)
    3 drops rosemary (*Rosmarinus officinalis*)
    2 drops mandarin (*Citrus reticulata*)

Coughs

Sometimes a cold can spread to the chest and cause a 'rattling' sound when the child breathes. Propping the child up can help, as can gently patting his back. The mucus should be encouraged to flow and not be suppressed in any way.

Treatment
- Vaporization
- Chest massage
- Application
- Recommended carriers: hypericum, sunflower, white lotion
- Recommended essential oils: cedarwood, *Eucalyptus smithii*, lavender (for spasmodic coughs), marjoram (sweet), rosemary, sandalwood, thyme (sweet)

Suggested Recipe
- Chest rub:
    - 20 ml hypericum (St John's wort)
    - 30 ml sunflower **or** 50 ml white lotion
    - 3 drops sandalwood (*Santalum album*)
    - 2 drops marjoram (sweet) (*Origanum majorana*)
    - 2 drops thyme (sweet) (*Thymus vulgaris* alcohol chemotype)

Cradle Cap

This is a type of eczema (seborrhoeic type) that is very common in young babies and children who have begun to have a head of hair. The scalp becomes crusty with yellow/white-coloured scales which do not usually cause any distress to the child. It is made worse by poor shampooing techniques and inadequate rinsing. Always use a mild shampoo, massage gently and rinse very thoroughly.

Treatment
- Massage
- Recommended carriers: olive, sweet almond
- Recommended essential oils: cedarwood, lavender*, rosemary, sandalwood*

Suggested Recipe
- Massage oil:
    20 ml olive
    30 ml sweet almond
    4 drops cedarwood (*Cedrus atlantica*)
    4 drops sandalwood (*Santalum album*)
    To be applied to scalp, massaged in well and left on overnight.
    Rub scales off when washing the hair next morning.

Croup

Croup is an acute infection of the larynx, most common in children under five years old. The symptoms are a harsh barking cough and grunting during breathing; usually the child also has a runny nose. Croup in its milder forms is often difficult to distinguish from a common cough and cold. However, in its more serious forms, shortness of breath and breathing difficulties make the croup apparent. Most cases of croup are mild, although the symptoms can be alarming. Always consult a doctor in any case of breathing difficulties.

Treatment
- Application – to neck and chest
- Inhalation – from a tissue (*see Chapter 4*)
- Vaporization – in conjunction with plenty of steam generated from a bowl of hot water or wet towels placed on a hot radiator (unless your child is asthmatic)
- Tepid bath – for reducing temperature
- Recommended carrier: white lotion
- Recommended essential oils: *Eucalyptus smithii*, marjoram (sweet), rosewood[*], sandalwood, thyme (sweet)

Suggested Recipes
- Inhalation mix for vaporization or tissue:
    2 drops *Eucalyptus smithii*
    1 drop marjoram (sweet) (*Origanum majorana*)
    1 drop rosewood (*Aniba rosaeodora*)

Crying

Although crying in itself is not an illness, constant crying can be a sign that your baby is unwell. It could also mean he is hungry, thirsty, wants his nappy changed, is bored, has colic, is teething, is too hot or cold or just wants your attention. Some babies cry for no apparent reason, although diet is always worth looking at. One youngster, after much effort to discover the cause, turned out to have a sensitivity to gluten. When this was removed from his diet, there was no more crying. It may not always be gluten, but in a case where there is asthma or eczema in the family, gluten and dairy products
(cow's milk, cheese) are the two usual offenders.

Treatment
- Bath
- Massage
- Recommended carrier: lime blossom
- Recommended essential oils: chamomile (Roman), cypress, frankincense, geranium, lavender, rose otto, ylang ylang

See also possible related ailments – such as **Colic**

Suggested Recipe
- Massage oil:
    40 ml grapeseed
    10 ml lime blossom
    3 drops frankincense (*Boswellia carteri*)
    2 drops chamomile (Roman) (*Chamaemelum nobile*)
    2 drops rose otto (*Rosa damascena*)

Cuts (and small wounds)

Small cuts and wounds can be treated as easily and efficiently with aromatherapy as with patented products; both have antiseptic properties.

Treatment
- Application:
- Initial application can be 1 drop of one of the suggested oils directly onto the cut, after which an application lotion should be used.

- Recommended carriers: calendula, hypericum, rose hip, white lotion
- Recommended essential oils: bergamot, chamomile (Roman), geranium, lavender, rosemary, rose otto, tea tree

Suggested Recipe
- Lotion:
    5 ml white lotion (in an egg cup)
    2 drops geranium (*Pelargonium graveolens*)
    2 drops lavender (*Lavandula angustifolia*)

Cystitis

This is an infection of the bladder, ureter and urethra. It causes a burning sensation when urine is passed and, because the bladder is made irritable by the condition, frequency of urination is marked. It is more common in girls than boys and can sometimes be caused by wiping the bottom from the anus towards the vulva.

Treatment
- Bath
- Recommended essential oils: cedarwood, *Eucalyptus smithii*, sandalwood, thyme (sweet)

Suggested Recipe
- Bath:
    2 drops sandalwood (*Santalum album*)
    1 drop cedarwood (*Cedrus atlantica*)
    1 drop *E. smithii*

Diarrhoea

This is the frequent passing of loose watery stools, which are often foul smelling and of an unusual colour such as greenish brown or yellow. Give plenty of fluids to guard against dehydration and, if accompanied by vomiting, consult the doctor – he or she will most likely give you hydrating and electrolyte-replacing drink powders for your child. Try to note the food eaten prior to diarrhoea in case of food sensitization; it could be the result of poorly cooked food or food that was incorrectly defrosted.

Treatment
- Fluids (give plenty of liquid to drink)
- Massage
- Recommended carriers: calendula, sunflower, white lotion
- Recommended essential oils: chamomile (Roman), geranium, ginger, lemon, marjoram (sweet), rosemary, sandalwood

Suggested Recipe
- Abdomen massage oil:
    - 10 ml calendula
    - 40 ml sunflower
    - 4 drops ginger (*Zingiber officinale*)
    - 4 drops rosemary (*Rosmarinus officinalis*)

Earache

Earache can be triggered by a number of different problems like mumps, measles, toothache, sinus congestion or an actual ear infection such as *otitis media*. A baby will normally cry shrilly and refuse to be comforted. The outer ear may be red and sometimes a discharge is visible (in which case a doctor should be consulted).

Treatment
- If connected to a cough or related problem, treat in conjunction with that condition
- Massage around outer ear – particularly immediately behind the ears
- Recommended carriers: hypericum, sweet almond, white lotion
- Recommended essential oils: chamomile (Roman), lavender, tea tree, thyme (sweet)

Suggested Recipe
- Massage oil:
    - 10 ml hypericum (St John's wort)
    - 40 ml sweet almond **or** white lotion
    - 4 drops lavender (*Lavandula angustifolia*)
    - 2 drops chamomile (Roman) (*Chamaemelum nobile*)
    - 2 drops tea tree (*Melaleuca alternifolia*)

Eczema

Infantile eczema is most common in young babies where there is asthma or hayfever in the family. (The three are connected and can be hereditary). It generally shows itself as raised, red scaly patches on the cheeks, behind the ears and where there are skin folds on the body, as in neck creases, elbows and knees. Some types of nappy rash, in an eczema-prone child, are more likely to respond to an eczema treatment than a normal barrier antiseptic cream.

A baby with eczema should never wear wool next to his skin – always use cotton or 50/50 cotton/polyester.

Seborrhoeic eczema (**Cradle Cap** – *see page 96*) can spread from the scalp to the forehead, eyebrows, cheeks and behind the ears. This is a more yellow, crusty type of eczema which can be softened with oil and gently removed to leave thin, pink skin behind (*see Chapter 6*).[2] Always protect this skin with the application of a carrier lotion with essential oils chosen from the list below until it has regained normal skin texture.

Although not well publicized, a change in diet can dramatically improve or worsen eczema, the usual offenders being dairy produce (cow's milk and cheese), wheat, and white, refined products (bread, sugar, etc.). When beginning serious treatment for eczema, diet *must* be investigated thoroughly and changed accordingly.

Treatment
- Bath
- Massage
- Body lotion
- Recommended carriers: avocado, calendula, carrot, sweet almond, rose hip, white lotion
- Recommended essential oils: bergamot, cedarwood, chamomile (Roman), frankincense*, geranium, lavender, rose otto, sandalwood, thyme (sweet)

Suggested Recipes
- Massage oil:
    - 30 ml sweet almond
    - 10 ml carrot

10 ml calendula
3 drops geranium (*Pelargonium graveolens*)
3 drops lavender (*Lavandula angustifolia*)
2 drops bergamot (*Citrus bergamia*)
- Application lotion:
30 ml white lotion
20 ml carrot
3 drops geranium (*Pelargonium graveolens*)
3 drops lavender (*Lavandula angustifolia*)
2 drops bergamot (*Citrus bergamia*)

Epilepsy

We do not presume to suggest treatment for epilepsy within these pages, but to offer a precautionary note. Massage, if done very, very gently on small areas of the body, can help relieve the stress of epilepsy. Do not massage the entire body on the first treatment, but build up gradually, perhaps starting only with the back. The massage must be non-stimulating, so keep all movements slow and gentle. Essential oils for stress can be used, perhaps the most useful being mandarin (*Citrus reticulata*) and rose otto (*Rosa damascena*).

Gastro-enteritis

This is an attack of vomiting together with diarrhoea and can cause repeated sharp abdominal pains and fever. It is usually caused by bacteria.

Treatment
- Vaporization
- Application
- Massage
- Recommended carriers: calendula, sunflower, white lotion
- Recommended essential oils: geranium, ginger, mandarin*, marjoram (sweet)

Suggested Recipe
Abdomen massage oil:
10 ml calendula
40 ml sunflower
4 drops ginger (*Zingiber officinale*)
4 drops mandarin (*Citrus reticulata*)

Hayfever (allergic rhinitis)

Not common in babies and usually only then in families who have a history of hayfever, eczema or asthma. Symptoms of hayfever include itchy, sensitive eyes, constant running nose, dry, chesty cough, headaches and a general feeling of lethargy.

Treatment
- Vaporization
- Inhalation
- Bath
- Face and chest lotion
- Recommended carriers: grapeseed, white lotion
- Recommended essential oils: *Eucalyptus smithii* *, rosewood*

Suggested Recipe
- Oils for vaporizer:
    2 drops *Eucalyptus smithii*
    2 drops rosewood (*Aniba rosaeodora*)

High Temperature

This can include fever or other ailments such as **Chicken pox, Influenza, Measles** (*see relevant sections in this chapter and Chapter 7*).

Treatment
(for lowering temperature)
- Tepid bath
- Recommended essential oil: *Eucalyptus smithii*

Suggested Recipe
- Bath:
    3 drops *Eucalyptus smithii*

Hyperactivity

Not many children are truly hyperactive, most children being simply extremely energetic! It has been said that if an experienced athlete were to follow a toddler around all day he or she would feel exhausted by bedtime (we know how that feels!). However, if your child is truly hyperactive, then diet is the first avenue to explore. Many colourings (e.g. orange squash, highly coloured sweets, etc.) and refined, bleached foods can be the direct cause of hyperactivity, and these therefore need to be excluded from your child's diet. Massage is the best way of calming the child – if you can catch him! Having treated several hyperactive children we would advise starting with massage of the hands only – more than that will bore the child and he will fidget. After a time, include the legs, then move to the back; gradually you will be able to build up to a full massage – if needed.

Treatment
- Vaporization
- Bath
- Massage
- Recommended carriers: lime blossom, sunflower
- Recommended essential oils: bergamot, chamomile (Roman), frankincense, geranium, lavender, mandarin, marjoram (sweet), rose otto, sandalwood, thyme (sweet), ylang ylang

Suggested Recipe
- Bath:
    2 drops sandalwood (*Santalum album*)
    1 drop frankincense (*Boswellia carteri*)
    1 drop ylang ylang (*Cananga odorata*)

Impetigo

This is a very contagious skin infection caused by bacteria. It usually appears first on the face as bright red spots, which turn into pustules containing a yellow pus. This fluid oozes out of the skin and then the spots dry to a crusty formation. Since it is so contagious all flannels, towels, bedding, etc. should be boiled and kept for the infected child's own use. Scratching must be discouraged because of the risk of scarring. The rash will spread from the face down the chest and sometimes to the lower body. It commonly appears after a cold, and eczema-prone children are more susceptible.[3]

Treatment
- Bath
- Massage
- Lotion application
- Recommended carriers: calendula, carrot, hypericum, white lotion
- Recommended essential oils: geranium, rosewood*, tea tree

Suggested Recipe
- Body lotion:
  50 ml white lotion
  4 drops geranium (*Pelargonium graveolens*)
  2 drops rosewood (*Aniba rosaeodora*)
  2 drops tea tree (*Melaleuca alternifolia*)

Insect Bites

Insect bites are hot to the touch, red and raised and can cause severe skin irritation.

Treatment
- Application
- Recommended carriers: carrot, olive, white lotion
- Recommended essential oils: chamomile (Roman), lavender, lemon, sandalwood, tea tree

Suggested Recipe
- Initially, any one of the essential oils listed above (whichever is nearest to hand), followed by:
- Application lotion:
  5 ml olive oil or white lotion
  2 drops chamomile (Roman) (*Chamaemelum nobile*)
  2 drops lavender (*Lavandula angustifolia*)

Insomnia

There's nothing quite as exhausting as having to wake up in the night to look after a sleepless child! There can be many reasons why a child will wake in the night and all of these should be checked out as well as giving aromatherapy treatment. Here is a checklist:

Is your child too hot in bed?
Too cold?
Hungry?
Does he have a blocked nose, cough or any other physical discomfort?
Does he wake to use the toilet?
Is it a habit?

Usually a warm bath at bedtime using oils such as sandalwood, ylang ylang or marjoram (sweet) can be very helpful. Also, put some oils onto a tissue to tuck under his pillowcase for inhalation. If your child is usually lively and energetic, a massage after his evening bath is a gentle way to relax and soothe him and encourage sleep. Lavender, if not the genuine oil, or if used in excess, can cause wakefulness, so always use only 1 or 2 drops (maximum) for children.

Treatment
- Application
- Bath
- Inhalation
- Massage
- Recommended carriers: lime blossom, sunflower, white lotion
- Recommended essential oils: bergamot, chamomile (Roman), lavender, lemon, mandarin, marjoram (sweet), sandalwood, ylang ylang

Suggested Recipe
30 ml lime blossom oil
20 ml sunflower oil
3 drops chamomile (Roman) (*Chamaemelum nobile*)
3 drops ylang ylang (*Cananga odorata*)
2 drops marjoram (sweet) (*Origanum majorana*)

Jaundice

Not an ailment, but a symptom of the build-up of bilirubin (a yellow pigment usually broken down by the liver) in the blood. Generally most common in newborn babies, who are then usually treated by ultra-violet light (which helps bilirubin to break down).[4] Other symptoms include yellowing eye-whites, nausea and putty-coloured stools.

Treatment
- Gentle massage in conjunction with UVA light treatment. Do not apply essential oil mixture immediately prior to UVA treatment – at least 30 minutes beforehand or any time afterwards is to be preferred.
- Recommended carrier: white lotion
- Recommended essential oils: geranium, lemon, mandarin, rosemary

Suggested Recipe
30 ml white lotion
4 drops lemon (*Citrus limon*)
2 drops geranium (*Pelargonium graveolens*)
2 drops mandarin (*Citrus reticulata*)

Lice

These small parasites jump from head to head and appear to like clean hair the best! They lay their small white eggs on the hair shaft, where they are firmly glued in position. The adults cause itching and an unpleasant tickling sensation as they move through the hair.

Treatment
- Recommended carrier: water
- Recommended essential oils: *Eucalyptus smithii*, rosemary, tea tree, thyme (sweet)*

Suggested Recipe
- Hair rinse:
    300 ml (½ pint) water
    2 drops *Eucalyptus smithii*
    2 drops rosemary (*Rosmarinus officinalis*)
    1 drop tea tree (*Melaleuca alternifolia*)

- Wash and rinse hair thoroughly. Use essential oils in the final rinse and towel dry – do not rinse out. Comb through and dry hair completely in the normal manner.

Measles

Measles usually starts with cold symptoms, a dry cough and a high temperature. White spots can be found inside the cheeks during the first few days. After a time, small red spots appear behind the ears and spread to the cheeks and over the body. Measles can have many complications, so always consult a doctor.

Treatment
- Bath
- Lotion application
- Recommended carriers: carrot (for inflammation), white lotion
- Recommended essential oils: cypress, *Eucalyptus smithii*, geranium, ginger, lavender, lemon*, marjoram (sweet), rosemary

Suggested Recipe
- Bath:
    2 drops lavender (*Lavandula angustifolia*)
    1 drop geranium (*Pelargonium graveolens*)
    1 drop lemon (*Citrus limon*)

Mouth Ulcers

Mouth ulcers can be triggered by a sugary diet, sharp-edged sweets, or by an allergy, infection or the herpes simplex virus. They are small, white, raised spots that usually do not stay long and go of their own accord.

Treatment
- Mouth wash
- Recommended carrier: water
- Recommended essential oils: bergamot, geranium, orange (sweet), rose otto, tea tree (for infection)

Suggested Recipe
- Mouth wash:
- 150 ml (½ cup) tepid boiled water
    1 drop orange (sweet) (*Citrus aurantium* var. *sinensis*)
    1 drop tea tree (*Melaleuca alternifolia*)

Nappy Rash

Nappy rash is really a type of contact dermatitis where the baby's skin is irritated by the urine and stools in the nappy. It can sometimes be eczema-induced.

It can also be due to a fungus (*see* **Thrush**). This is when the red spotting is pinpointed and does not respond to ordinary treatment for nappy rash.

In all cases, change nappies frequently and try to keep the nappy loose enough to allow air to circulate. Leave the nappy off for several short periods throughout the day. Make sure that towelling nappies are thoroughly rinsed through to remove all traces of washing powder (which can cause or increase the irritation). We recommend using disposable nappies for helping with persistent nappy rash.

Treatment
- Bath
- Massage
- Lotion application
- Recommended carriers: calendula, carrot, sunflower, white lotion
- Recommended essential oils:
    for dermatitis – bergamot, chamomile (Roman), frankincense*, geranium, lavender, sandalwood
    for eczema – chamomile (Roman), geranium, lavender, rose otto
    for thrush – *see* **Thrush**

Suggested Recipe
(dermatitis type)
- Massage oil:
    20 ml calendula
    30 ml white lotion

3 drops frankincense (*Boswellia carteri*)
3 drops lavender (*Lavandula angustifolia*)
2 drops geranium (*Pelargonium graveolens*)

Nosebleeds

These can be a result of a knock or fall, or may accompany a heavy cold; they can occasionally be stress-induced.

Treatment
- Compress
- Application lotion
- Recommended carriers: water, white lotion
- Recommended essential oils: cypress, lemon
- Put a large key or other cold metal object inside the back of the child's clothes. Apply cypress lotion directly on forehead and nose, or use a compress.

Suggested Recipe
    5 ml white lotion
    2 drops cypress (*Cupressus sempervirens*)
    2 drops lemon (*Citrus limon*)

Rashes

Rashes can be caused by eczema, allergies or heat. Also, infectious diseases can sometimes be accompanied by a rash. We will deal here with heat rash (*see also* **Allergies** and **Eczema**).

Heat rash usually occurs when the baby is wrapped up too warmly, or when there is no suitable shade on a hot day. Many parents mistakenly think that newborn babies need to be wrapped up in several shawls on top of the nappy and other baby clothes. This can be quite dangerous, as babies are not able to remove the extra layers of clothing themselves and it can lead, in extreme cases, to overheating and suffocation. Usually, if *you* feel warm enough, your baby is warm enough.

Babies and young children also need protection from the sun, as overexposure to the sun can cause a rash on delicate skin (*see* **Sunburn**).

As a rule, heat rash displays itself as crops of tiny red blotches, usually appearing in areas where there is concentrated heat: the nappy area, under the arms, the folds of the neck, the abdomen, etc.

Treatment
- Bath
- Lotion application
- Recommended carriers: calendula, white lotion
- Recommended essential oils: chamomile (Roman), lavender, rose otto, sandalwood

Suggested Recipe
- Bath:
    2 drops chamomile (Roman) (*Chamaemelum nobile*)
    1 drop lavender (*Lavandula angustifolia*)
    1 drop sandalwood (*Santalum album*)

Ringworm

Ringworm is caused by a fungal infection and not a worm at all! It is infectious between humans and animals. The infection causes red scaly circular patches which are clear in the centre. It can cause hair loss on the body and, more noticeably, on the scalp. It can also infect the nails, where treatment takes a long time – as long, in fact, as it takes the nail to grow completely out. However, the area will eventually clear.

Treatment
- Bath
- Lotion application
- Recommended carrier: white lotion
- Recommended essential oils: geranium, rose otto*, tea tree, thyme (sweet)

Suggested Recipe
- Application lotion:
    50 ml white lotion
    4 drops tea tree (*Melaleuca alternifolia*)
    2 drops geranium (*Pelargonium graveolens*)
    2 drops thyme (sweet) (*Thymus vulgaris* linalool or geraniol chemotype)

Scabies

Scabies is when tiny mites enter the skin and lay eggs under the surface of the skin. The eggs, when hatched, crawl to the surface and begin the process all over again. It is generally a very irritating rash, producing red lines across the skin which may bleed and become inflamed when scratched. Scabies generally appears between the toes and fingers, and in the groin and buttock creases.

Treatment
- Bath
- Lotion application
- Recommended carrier: white lotion
- Recommended essential oils: chamomile (Roman), lemon*, rosewood, tea tree, thyme (sweet)

Suggested Recipe
- Bath:
      2 drops thyme (sweet) (*Thymus vulgaris* linalool or geraniol chemotype)
      1 drop rosewood (*Aniba rosaeodora*)
      1 drop tea tree (*Melaleuca alternifolia*)

Sleeplessness

See **Insomnia**

Sunburn

Children exposed to strong sunlight for relatively long periods of time are easily burnt by the sun. When in prams and buggies children should *always* have protection, particularly around the head, although ideally all exposed skin should be covered up most of the time.

Sunburn can be very painful and hot, and in severe cases can cause peeling and blistering. The child can feel sick and confused. If your child is sick, confused and unable to keep his balance, this is likely to be the more serious condition known as *sunstroke* – in which case a doctor should be consulted.

Treatment
(for sunburn, not sunstroke)
- Bath
- Lotion application
- Recommended carriers: carrot, rose hip, white lotion
- Recommended essential oils: lavender, rose otto, sandalwood

Suggested Recipe
- Lotion application:
    50 ml white lotion
    4 drops lavender (*Lavandula angustifolia*)
    2 drops rose otto (*Rosa damascena*)
    2 drops sandalwood (*Santalum album*)

Teething (Toothache in Children)

Lots of babies seem to suffer mild discomfort during the natural process of
teething. These symptoms can include: red flushed cheeks, slight temperature,
runny nose, red, sore gums and irritability. Check first that these symptoms
are not caused by anything more serious which needs medical attention.

Treatment
- Lotion application
- Recommended carriers: hypericum, white lotion
- Recommended essential oils: chamomile (Roman), ginger, lavender,
  marjoram (sweet), tea tree
- A very small amount of your chosen mixture can be applied twice a day with
  your fingertip over the affected area of gum and on the outside cheek area.

Suggested Recipe
- Lotion application:
    30 ml white lotion
    20 ml hypericum
    4 drops chamomile (Roman) (*Chamaemelum nobile*)
    2 drops lavender (*Lavandula angustifolia*)
    2 drops marjoram (sweet) (*Origanum majorana*)

Temper Tantrums

Not strictly speaking an 'ailment', though it seems like a crisis at the time –
especially if it is in the supermarket on a busy day! Regular tantrums need
regular attention. This means spending some time every day talking to your
child, perhaps massaging his back or hands and generally defusing any stress
build-up between you. If your child is unable to talk to you because he is too
young, this does not mean he will not recognize a soothing tone in your voice.
Bathing together with essential oils is relaxing – and keeping a tissue with
the same oils on it in a plastic bag in your coat pocket can then work in the
supermarket. Your child will associate the 'nice' smell with moments spent
in harmony with you.

Treatment
- Inhalation
- Bath
- Massage
- Recommended carrier: lime blossom
- Recommended essential oils: lavender, mandarin, rose otto, sandalwood,
  ylang ylang

Suggested Recipe
- Bath:
      2 drops mandarin (*Citrus reticulata*)
      2 drops ylang ylang (*Cananga odorata*)

Threadworms

Threadworms are very common in children. The eggs are picked up and
become lodged under the fingernails. When the child puts his fingers in his
mouth the eggs enter the digestive tract and hatch. The newly-hatched worms
then travel the full length of the intestinal tract and emerge at the other end.
These worms then lay their eggs around the child's anus. This causes intense
itching, the child scratches his bottom, the eggs lodge under the nails, the
fingers go in the mouth and the whole process starts again.

This is one of the reasons why it is always important for people to wash their
hands thoroughly and dry them on a clean towel after each visit to the toilet.

Parents can also 'catch' the worms from their children if hygiene is not observed in the home.

Treatment
- Bath
- Lotion application (to be applied to the anal area and hands)
- Recommended carrier: white lotion
- Recommended essential oils: chamomile (Roman) (for itching), *Eucalyptus smithii* *, lavender (for itching), tea tree, thyme (sweet)

Suggested Recipe
- Bath:
    2 drops *Eucalyptus smithii*
    1 drop tea tree (*Melaleuca alternifolia*)
    1 drop thyme (sweet) (*Thymus vulgaris*)

Throat Infections

A sore throat often accompanies the common cold, fever, chest conditions and many other childhood illnesses. Tonsillitis, where the tonsils are inflamed due to bacterial infection, is common in children. It can be detected easily by noting the enlarged tonsils, which are reddened and often covered in white spots.

Treatment
- Lotion application (throat and chest)
- Gargle – *see page 75*
- Recommended carrier: white lotion
- Recommended essential oils: lavender, sandalwood, tea tree, thyme (sweet)

Suggested Recipe
- Lotion application:
    50 ml white lotion
    3 drops tea tree (*Melaleuca alternifolia*)
    2 drops lavender (*Lavandula angustifolia*)
    2 drops sandalwood (*Santalum album*)
    2 drops thyme (sweet) (*Thymus vulgaris* linalool or geraniol chemotype)

Thrush

Thrush is a fungal infection affecting the digestive system. In babies it is most common in the mouth, looking like white curds on the tongue and inside of the cheeks. If this is not treated at an early stage, the fungus can reach the bottom, causing nappy rash (which looks like little red pinheads – *see page 109*). Dummies and bottles and all feeding equipment must be carefully sterilized.

Treatment
- Bath
- Massage (nappy area)
- Recommended carriers: calendula, sunflower, white lotion (for bottom)
- Recommended essential oils: geranium, lavender, lemon, rosewood, tea tree, thyme (sweet)

N.B. You can make an effective anti-bacterial cleansing fluid from 600 ml (1 pint) of cooled boiled water and 5 drops of tea tree (*Melaleuca alternifolia*). Shake well together in a screw-top container and leave dummies, etc. in the fluid for 30 minutes. Rinse well before use.

Suggested Recipe
- Lotion application:
    20 ml calendula
    30 ml white lotion
    3 drops lavender (*Lavandula angustifolia*)
    3 drops rosewood (*Aniba rosaeodora*)
    2 drops tea tree (*Melaleuca alternifolia*)

- Massage oil:
    10 ml calendula oil
    40 ml sunflower oil
    2 drops chamomile (Roman) (*Chamaemelum nobile*)
    2 drops lemon (*Citrus limon*)
    2 drops tea tree (*Melaleuca alternifolia*)
    2 drops thyme (sweet) (*Thymus vulgaris* linalool or geraniol chemotype)

Tonsillitis

See Throat Infections

Travel Sickness

Children are often travel sick, the first symptoms being a pallid colour, accompanied by the child being unusually quiet and perhaps experiencing nausea, dizziness, headaches and fatigue. Diet can help here by giving the child a light protein meal before the journey and limiting fizzy drinks. Chocolate and sweets must also be avoided. Pack plenty of toys to keep your child busy and less aware of the motion of the car or bus. We have found wrist bands to be helpful too (available from Seaband UK – *see Useful Addresses*).

Treatment
- Inhalation
- Lotion application (before journey)
- Recommended carrier: white lotion
- Recommended essential oils: bergamot, chamomile (Roman), ginger, lemon, orange (sweet), rosewood*, sandalwood*

Suggested Recipe
- Inhalation (from a tissue):
    2 drops orange (sweet) (*Citrus aurantium* var. *sinensis*)
    1 drop bergamot (*Citrus bergamia*)
    1 drop ginger (*Zingiber officinale*)

Verrucae

Verrucae are warts on the soles of the feet and are due to a viral infection, usually picked up from the swimming baths or by walking barefoot on dirty carpets. They can also be caught by bathing or swapping shoes with an infected child. The verrucae are painful to stand on and yet look surprisingly small from the outside. This is because they grow upwards into the fleshy part of the foot.

Treatment
- Massage
- Direct application
- Foot bath
- Lotion
- Recommended carrier: white lotion
- Recommended essential oils: bergamot, geranium*, lemon, thyme (sweet)

Suggested Recipes
- Direct application:
    2 drops lemon (*Citrus limon*) (on cotton bud)
- Foot bath:
    2 drops thyme (sweet) (*Thymus vulgaris* linalool or geraniol chemotype)
    1 drop geranium (*Pelargonium graveolens*)
    1 drop lemon (*Citrus limon*)
- Lotion application:
    1 tsp white lotion
    2 drops lemon (*Citrus limon*)
    2 drops thyme (sweet) (*Thymus vulgaris* linalool or geraniol chemotype)

Vomiting

Sometimes due to over-eating or over-excitement, but can accompany some infectious diseases.

Treatment
- Inhalation
- Bath
- Application lotion (abdomen)
- Recommended essential oils: bergamot, chamomile (Roman), ginger, lemon, orange (sweet), rosewood, sandalwood

Suggested Recipe
    50 ml white lotion
    4 drops ginger (*Zingiber officinale*)
    2 drops orange (sweet) (*Citrus aurantium* var. *sinensis*)
    2 drops rosewood (*Aniba rosaeodora*)

Warts

Warts can present themselves anywhere on the body. They can look like small cabbages, flat brown moles, or verrucae. Warts are caused by a viral infection.

Treatment
- Direct application
- Hand bath
- Lotion
- Recommended carrier: white lotion
- Recommended essential oils: bergamot, geranium*, lemon, thyme (sweet)

Suggested Recipes
- Direct application:
    2 drops lemon (*Citrus limon*) (on cotton bud)
- Hand bath:
    2 drops thyme (sweet) (*Thymus vulgaris* linalool or geraniol chemotype)
    1 drop geranium (*Pelargonium graveolens*)
    1 drop lemon (*Citrus limon*)
- Lotion application:
    1 tsp white lotion
    2 drops lemon (*Citrus limon*)
    2 drops thyme (sweet) (*Thymus vulgaris* linalool or geraniol chemotype)

1 *A – Z of Childhood Ailments* (Bounty Press, 1992)
2 As above
3 As above
4 As above

6

Massage

The benefits of massage to babies and children cannot be extolled high enough! Massage is touch in its most positive form, and most children love being held and cuddled by a parent. Let us look at the areas where massage can help.

1. Parent/Child Bonding

Unfortunately, parenting often comes as rather a surprise to many new mothers and fathers, when 'bonding' is not always a natural process and has to be worked at (like most relationships in life). Learning to massage your child can be an important building block in this process, whereby even a mechanical massage routine can lead to genuine empathy and love between parent and child.

2. Security

Once a child is used to a massage routine and it becomes part of a daily or weekly procedure, then she will associate the massage with a parent's total attention, and recognize it as a valuable gift of love.

3. Confidence

Although it seems a long way away, one day your child will grow up! Too many teenagers are self-conscious about their bodies. In today's world young adults are bombarded with 'the perfect body image', which can lead to feelings of inadequacy about their own size or shape. Shyness is also a problem in teenage years.

We believe that massage from an early age (although it is never too late to start) can nurture feelings of confidence and a positive self-image. Children can learn to look at their bodies in a more confident way and be 'in touch' with themselves as well as relaxed. It also helps if siblings are taught to *give* massage as well as receive it, as our own children do. Penny has found that, with her own children, giving as well as receiving encourages harmony and tolerance in the household and a certain degree of respect for each other. This is an especially effective treatment for warring brothers! A simple back massage is usually sufficient, and does not cause embarrassment between siblings of different genders.

4. As a Prophylactic

It is generally accepted that stress is responsible for a great number of emotional and physical problems. Regular massage will help to dissipate stress and at the same time improve circulation and muscle tone (massage is a form of passive exercise). Essential oils when combined with massage enhance these benefits; they also have a strong role to play as preventatives.

5. Emotional and Physical Benefits of Massage

As already mentioned, the early emotional benefits gained by massage include security, love, comfort and stability. Different races from all over the world behave differently from each other. You are sure to have noticed that Mediterranean people are much more likely to hug and greet each other physically than are English people. We believe that this is an advantage and helps children and adults to feel secure and comfortable in their environment.

The later benefits of massage are also very marked and can be divided into two sections:

1) Emotional

Through massage children can learn to love themselves. They appreciate their bodies and they grow up unashamed of them. This leads to self-confidence and helps them to be at ease with others. Massage from a very early age can help to combat low self-esteem and encourage healthy self-love. Self-confidence, feeling at ease with others and being able to love yourself leads to a stress-free life with others.

Just imagine – if we did not wonder what other people thought of us; if only we did not have to compare ourselves with pictures in magazines; if only we were all comfortable with ourselves – what a wonderful place the world would be! This must be the ultimate aim for any parent: to bring up an emotionally secure and stable child.

2) Health Benefits

The health benefits of massage are numerous even without the added boon of essential oils. Massage increases lung capacity. In a study in a hospital on the south coast of England, it was shown that babies in incubators developed their lung capacity much more quickly if they were touched or stroked by their parents than if they were just handled by a nurse or left in their incubators.[1] This has been proved over and over again. A child can have nourishment, clothing and a place to sleep, but if she is not loved or spoken to or touched at all then she seems to give up the will to live.

Increased lung capacity is vital to the cellular health of the body, because the more oxygen a child can take in the better the cell regeneration – and therefore the better the health of the child.

A child will also benefit from smooth skin. Vegetable oil carriers are all very healing and nourishing to a developing skin and can encourage it to be not only smooth but also healthy. This leads to fewer skin problems in later life and can dramatically reduce existing ones such as psoriasis, eczema, dermatitis and acne.

Massage is wonderful for the nervous system. Many of our nerve endings are housed in the layers of the skin. You know from experience that if you bump yourself, rubbing the area will take away the pain; it therefore follows that the nervous system is affected by touch on the skin. It is also well known that massage is a wonderful aid for relieving stress in adults and is therefore equally effective on children, helping to calm them down when they are fractious, tired or hyperactive.

The digestive system is also affected by massage. Gentle massage on the abdomen can be very effective. However, it must be gentle and light, as there are no bones between the relative organs and the skin for protection. However, regular abdomen massage can help alleviate problems such as constipation, diarrhoea or nausea.

Another health benefit of massage is a healthy mind–body relationship, whereby the mind and body can help create a healthy developing child.

Other benefits include:

- relief of mental and physical fatigue; induces deep relaxation
- improved mobility; massage is a form of passive exercise
- promotion of easy and correct posture, therefore producing better health
- stimulation of body and mind without negative side-effects
- reduction of inflammation and/or pain
- improvement of the circulation of blood and lymph
- increase in the detoxifying function of the kidneys
- elimination via the lymphatic system.

From the above you can see that a prophylactic effect is gained by regular massage. This means that disease can be kept at bay just by keeping the body systems as healthy as possible with massage. Much can be achieved by giving up even five minutes of your time to massage your child; if she loves it, give her more time – 15 to 20 minutes is usually long enough for most children. It is beneficial if you let your child rest afterwards (covered with a blanket). She may even go to sleep; ours often do!

What Is Massage?

The word massage originally comes from a Greek word meaning 'to knead'. Massage is the manipulation of the soft tissues of the body, most effectively performed with the hands. There are many types of massage movements, of which we will describe some of the simplest and most useful, each used to produce different effects on the whole body.

Description of Massage Movements

1) Effleurage, or Stroking

Effleurage is carried out using the whole of the hand, with a constant upward pressure being applied in long smooth strokes, always directly towards the heart and with a light return back to the starting position. The rhythm and hand contact of this movement is intended to provide relaxation at the beginning and end of every section of massage performed on the body. Effleurage has a relaxing effect, increasing circulation and warming up the soft tissues of the body.

2) Frictions
With frictions the skin is moved over the underlying bones using circling movements, usually with the thumbs. When the thumbs have made circular movements over a limited area they are then lifted so that the hands and fingers can glide back to a position where the frictions can be repeated. The effects of frictions are to release tension, increase circulation and aid the elimination of waste products.

3) Kneading
This movement consists of grasping and releasing soft tissues of the body in a lifting, rolling or pressing movement, usually using all of the hand. Although the pressure is intermittent, the rhythm should remain constant.

These are just three types of massage movements. There is another type, which comes under the heading 'Percussion'. Percussion movements include tapping, slapping, hacking, pounding and beating, and are not thought to be suitable for use on children or for aromatherapy, where the main desired effect is to relieve stress and tension.

Preparation for Massage

1) The Room
The room should be warm and cosy. The child's body heat will drop during massage unless there is a heater in the room, it is a hot day or there are plenty of towels and blankets to cover her up.

The lighting must be soft and comforting (not fluorescent) so that the child is comfortable when lying on her back, looking at the ceiling. A bedside lamp is ideal.

Sometimes it helps you and your child to relax if there is some soft music playing. Many massage tapes are now available on the market and you could have fun choosing one together.

2) Yourself

Before massaging, remove any jewellery that may scratch your child.
Ensure that your nails are short and clean and that your hands are warm.

Try to avoid long-sleeved clothing, as this can trail across the body, causing a
tickling sensation. A sensible outfit would be a short-sleeved T-shirt tucked into
leggings or jogging pants. If you have long hair, tie it back away from your face.

Keep your hands flexible and relaxed. As you become more experienced in
massage you will become more conscious of the welfare of your hands. Using
gloves for gardening, washing up and peeling vegetables can help to keep your
hands smooth and in good condition. To increase flexibility in your hands,
practise squeezing a small rubber ball every day, one minute in each hand,
clenching your fingers as tightly as possible and then relaxing them. Do not
forget to remove any jewellery such as a watch or a ring with a large stone,
which may catch or scratch your child's skin.

3) Your Equipment

A massage couch, kitchen or dining table, or the floor (*see page 121*).

You will also need:

- an old sheet to protect the massage couch, table or floor area (*see page 126*)
- a pillow
- two bath towels
- a small blanket
- an egg-cup in which to put your massage oil, placed inside a bowl
  (to catch any drips of oil)
- a headband to keep your child's hair off her forehead (if necessary)
- a bedside lamp
- a tape and tape player
- a box of tissues (to wipe your hands)
- your prepared massage oil

4) Amount of Oil Used

It is important to use the right amount of oil to enable you to move smoothly –
but only just – over your child's body. If you can slide around easily – and the
body glistens – you have used too much oil.

The best way to learn how to use the right amount is to hold your fingers firmly against the bottle and tip the bottle against them. Apply this to your child or baby – and repeat until you have enough to move without slipperiness.

5) Your Child

Before massage your child should be relaxed and open about the whole idea. She needs to have emptied her bladder and have on her underwear (if she prefers this) – and a large towel. Making her comfortable before starting the massage is essential. The ideal time to massage is after a warm, relaxing bath.

6) Standing Properly

Incorrect posture will make you tired. How relaxed you are will in the end determine how relaxing your massage is. If you are standing in a free and easy relaxed manner with your feet about 45 cm (18 in) apart, then your body is able to move freely from your child's feet towards her head without undue strain on your back. Always bend your front knee when doing effleurage on a large area, aiming to move your body rather than relying on muscular strength.

Posture is obviously easiest if you have a massage couch. A massage couch is ideal because it is firm and of a height which will not harm your back and will enable you to apply the best possible pressure onto your child. However, if you do not have a massage bed there are two or three alternatives:

- *A bed*
  A bed, while being lovely for your child to lie on, is not ideal for massage. It is not a good height for your back and can in fact lead to you needing a massage! Apart from this it may be too soft.

- *The kitchen or dining table*
  This is preferable to using your child's bed, but you will need an activity mat, a folded duvet or a blanket under the protective sheet for her to lie on, as to lie on a table for any length of time can be quite uncomfortable.

- *The floor*
  The floor, which will also need an activity mat, a folded duvet or blanket under the protective sheet, is, like a table, better than using a bed. You can kneel, sitting on your haunches on the floor to give the massage. Obviously this is not as comfortable as using a table or a massage couch, nor is it good

for your posture, but it is the next best alternative. It is perhaps another good reason for doing part massage rather than a full body massage.

Before beginning massage you must always position yourself correctly as suggested above and make sure that most of your work comes from your lower back and legs (if standing). To do a massage from the shoulders, thinking of only your arms and hands, will lead to upper back tension and strain and will mean that your hands are not as 'floppy' as required for doing massage. There should be no tension in your hands whatsoever and very little in your arms, with the main thrust coming from your hips – letting your body movement either push your hands where you want them to go or allow them to return to the starting position (and not forgetting to bend your front knee). A massage done with relaxed hands and arms is much more pleasant to receive than one done with tense arms and hands – therefore your posture is very important.

7) Contact
Complete contact between your hands and your child's body is essential. This contact should never be broken. It is important that contact is maintained all the way during the massage of each part of the body – always keep one hand on the child throughout – this is reassuring to your child and maintains both continuity and a feeling of togetherness. Taking off both your hands halfway through massaging your child's back, for instance, will be very disruptive to her relaxation. It may also make you lose your place in the massage routine, which may therefore also disrupt you. If you need to blow your nose, or stop to see what to do next, remove only one hand, waiting at the beginning or end of the movement (not in the middle) until you are ready to re-commence. Do not worry about this – or about your massage not being 'technically correct' – the most important thing is to keep going and let your instincts guide you.

8) Pressure
Pressure is always important in massage, but is even more so when massaging children. It should not be too heavy – nor should it be too light. However, it is obvious that on a newborn baby the lighter the pressure, the better. As your child gets older you will find that your pressure will increase slightly.

It is important that you always make the main thrust of your movement towards the heart, returning from the heart without pressure. If it is not possible to get the whole of your hand on the part of your child's body you are massaging (for instance on a baby's leg) then use as much of the length of your fingers as possible, remembering to reduce your pressure accordingly, as fingers are bony and can be hard. Curve your hand or fingers around her leg.

9) Speed and Rhythm
Massage should generally be slow, gentle and rhythmical. This is the most relaxing for your child and more beneficial for her circulation. It can sometimes help to put on a restful music tape, which will not only help you to pace your massage accordingly but will have the added benefit of helping your child to relax.

10) State of Mind
The state of your mind is very important. If you are angry or feeling negative, rushed or irritable this will transfer itself to your child, so it is best not to massage her when you feel like this. It is very important not to do a massage in a hostile environment, as this will lead your child to think of massage as an unpleasant chore that you have to perform rather than as a gift of your own time which you want to give.

To prepare yourself for massage, sit down for five minutes first and listen to your favourite piece of music or a special relaxation tape, or just spend a couple of minutes talking to your child about something that relaxes both of you, such as a pleasant day out, etc.

Precautions with Massage

1) Recent Surgery
Never massage over areas of new scar tissue; always wait until the scar is no longer red and sore. However, lavender can be applied regularly to aid the healing of the scar.

2) Recent Fractures
If your child has had a recent fracture or break, wait at least two months before massaging the area. Oils can be used in the bath or applied gently to aid the healing process.

3) Cuts and Bruises

Take care if your child has cuts and bruises, ensuring that your pressure over these areas is always very light. If the cuts or bruises are large avoid the whole area, and treat instead with essential oils in the bath or gently applied in a lotion.

4) Infectious Diseases

It is not beneficial to massage a child who has a fever or is infectious, as she will be hot and aching. Treatment with oils in the bath is always preferable in such cases.

5) Medical Conditions

Conditions like epilepsy, heart conditions and other hereditary and medical problems do not preclude massage as long as care is taken. However, if your child is under the care of a doctor then ethically it is better to tell him or her that you are giving your child massage treatments.

If you are in doubt about whether or not to massage, do not guess; phone a qualified aromatherapist for advice (one who is a member of a professional association).

Children Massaging Others

Children love receiving massage. Many children who are used to being massaged regularly may often lie down and ask for it, so to receive it must be a wonderful thing. Also, after a massage, children take great delight and joy in massaging their parent's feet or hands – or shoulders – in return. They find just as much joy in giving as receiving, therefore this should be encouraged. It will also help them in later life if they are able both to receive and to give unconditionally.

We have found that allowing children to massage each other definitely helps friendly sibling relationships, whereby the children, instead of arguing, give each other a massage – creating a harmonious atmosphere. The children become more outgoing and less inhibited with each other in a safe context.

NB On a cautionary note here, although massage is encouraged between brothers and sisters and parents, we should not be naive when it comes to our children's relationships with outsiders and strangers. It should be made clear at all times to your children that massage is an activity which takes place within the family, and even then within strict boundaries of personal respect. We need to teach our children the difference between freedom in the home and freedom in society, which unfortunately in today's world are two very different things.

Baby Massage

Stage One

A new baby is a miracle! New mothers and fathers can often be seen cuddling, stroking, nuzzling, sniffing and sometimes even licking their new babies! This is massage in its most important early phase. Yet many parents will want to know 'how do I massage my baby?'

In our experience babies do not come straight from the womb expecting to have, or indeed, to enjoy a 'proper' massage.

First, they prefer to be swaddled or cuddled, and feel insecure being laid out flat for massage. Secondly, a new baby's skin is usually a couple of sizes too big and massaging such delicate 'baggy' skin is quite difficult. Massaging a new baby starts with caressing and fondling. We would recommend using an essential oil – perhaps one used in the labour ward – 1 drop on a tissue tucked into your bra. This way your baby becomes accustomed to a particular aroma from an early age. Penny used rose otto together with lavender for her four babies, keeping the tissue near her whenever they were fed or cuddled. Eventually, by putting the same oil on a tissue tucked under the corner of the cot sheet, she found that her children slept easily and were not so fretful in the night.

Stage Two

After getting to know your baby in the early days, you may then wish to think about using simple massage movements. The best way to start is by making yourself comfortable on a bed or settee, with your upper body supported by cushions or pillows. Put a flannelette sheet or soft towel over your abdomen and chest and lay the baby tummy down on your stomach. His head should be to one side, pointing towards your face. Apply a *very* small amount of your massage blend (*see Chapter 4*) on to your hands and warm the oil by rubbing your palms and fingers gently together. You are now ready for two simple 'introductory' massage movements:

1 Place your hands gently on your baby's buttocks, fingers pointing away from you. With *very* light pressure draw your hands towards you, bringing them gently up baby's back to the shoulder, ending on your fingertips (Figure 1). Very gently, using middle and ring fingers only, return down the sides of baby's body to the buttocks. Repeat several times.

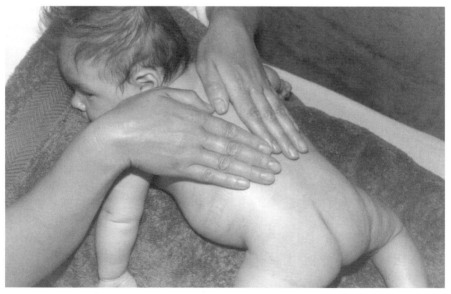

Figure 1

2 Turn baby over and draw your knees up towards you. Nestle baby, head away from you on your stomach, your knees supporting baby's head. With one hand, hold one of your baby's hands. This makes him feel secure and stops him 'thrashing' around. With your other hand gently place your finger lengths on baby's tummy. Draw clockwise circles around his navel, being as gentle as possible and using as much of the surface area of your fingers (and palm – if room) as you can (Figure 2).

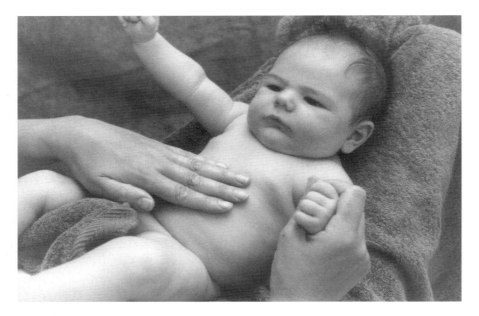

Figure 2

These two simple movements will be enough to start with, ensuring that your confidence and the baby's acceptance of the massage develop gently and slowly. Too much too soon may be wearing for mother, and perhaps upsetting for baby, so be patient. You and your baby are constantly learning together in a two-way process in which every action can produce an encouraging response such as a gurgle, coo or, later on, a smile.

Full Baby Massage

This is carried out with baby lying on a soft towel on the floor – in a warm room. Start with your baby lying face up.

Scalp

Place your fingertips on baby's scalp and very gently move the scalp over the bone (Figure 3). You will find this happens very easily on a newborn baby, as the skin on the scalp is quite loose and movable. Keep moving to a new area of the scalp and repeat the gentle scalp frictions. This movement helps to relax your baby and prepare him for further massage.

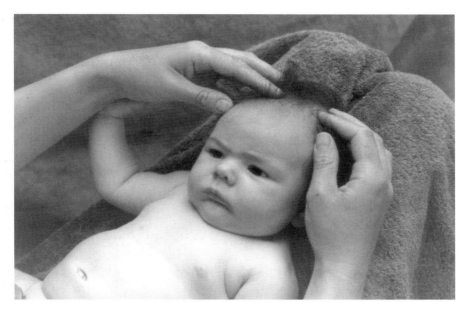

Figure 3

Tummy and Chest

Apply oil to baby's tummy.

1 Whole hand circling on abdomen
   Using one hand to hold one of baby's hands, place as much of your free hand
   as possible on his abdomen, gently moving it in a clockwise circle around
   your baby's navel. Take his chest into this movement also (Figure 4).
   Repeat two or three times.

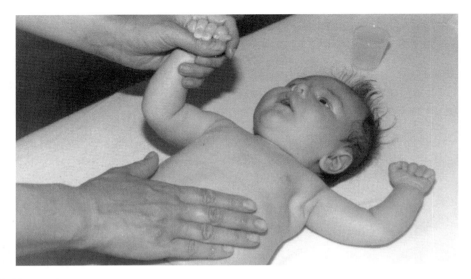

2 Butterfly movement
   Place the fingertips of both hands gently below your baby's tummy button.
   Move your hands gently up her abdomen to his shoulders, then sweep down
   gently underneath the rib cage at the sides of his body, and back to just
   below his navel (Figure 5). The pressure should be mainly on the upward
   movement but should be kept very, very light. Repeat two or three times.
3 Repeat movement 1 two to three times.

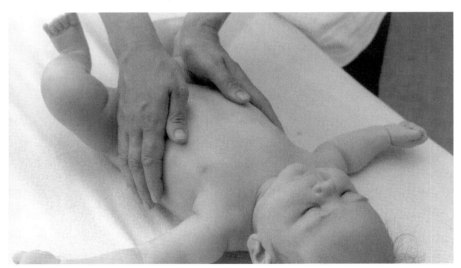

Foot and Leg Massage

Oil the front of your baby's legs and feet.

1 Foot massage
  Hold your baby's right foot with your left hand, fingers on top of his foot and thumb on his sole. Move your thumb in slow, gentle circles over the middle area of the sole of his foot (Figure 6).

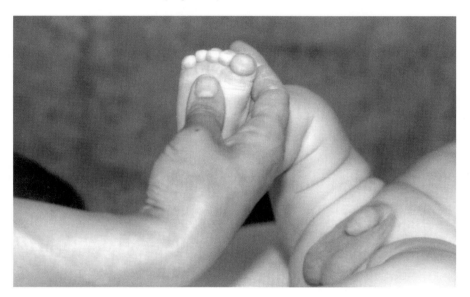

Figure 6

2 Circling up leg
  With your right hand holding your baby's foot, slowly circle up your baby's leg to his knee with your left thumb, starting at the ankle (Figure 7). On reaching his knee, gently slide back down to his ankle with your whole hand. Repeat two to three times.

Opposite: Figures 4 & 5

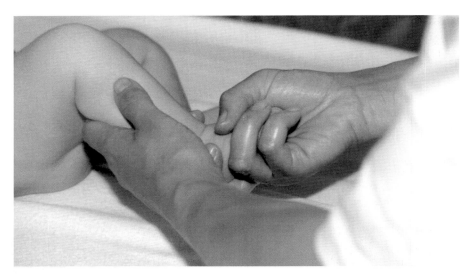

3 Effleurage of leg
   Still holding your baby's right leg, sweep your left hand (little finger leading)
   up to the top of his leg and return gently. As you go up, cover as much of his
   leg as possible, going up the shin bone, over the knee and right up to the
   groin area, gently sliding back down the outside of the leg (Figure 8).
   Repeat two to three times.

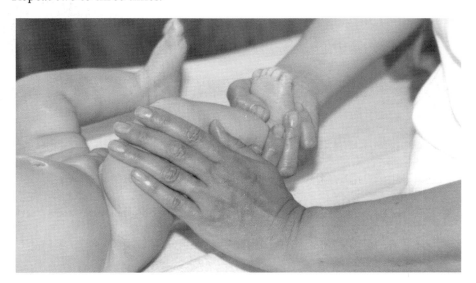

4 Repeat movement 1 on baby's foot.
5 Repeat movements 1 – 4 on your baby's left foot and leg, using your left hand
  to hold his left foot (your right hand will do the effleurage movement up the
  whole leg).

Arm and Hand Massage

Oil baby's arms and hands.

1 Hand massage
  Hold your baby's right fingers with your right hand and circle his palm
  with your left thumb in slow clockwise circles (Figure 9).

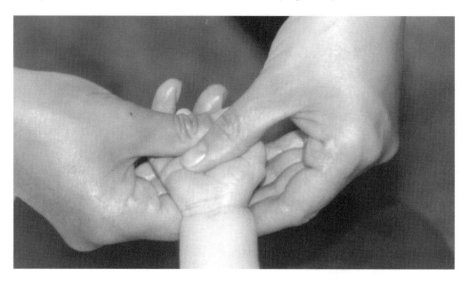

Figure 9

2 Effleurage of arm
  Holding your baby's right hand with your right hand, move very gently up
  his arm with your left hand, going up her forearm, over his elbow crease
  and reaching his shoulder (Figure 10). Circle around his shoulder and return
  gently on the back of his arm. Repeat two to three times.

Opposite: *Figures 7 & 8*

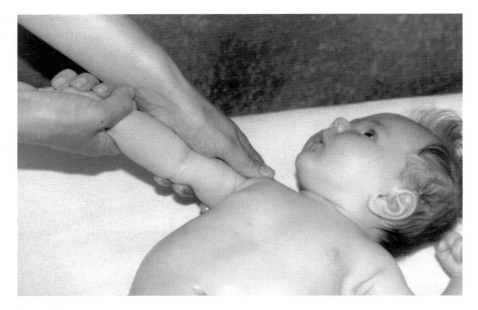

Figure 10

3 Repeat both movements on your baby's left arm, changing your holding and
   active hand to match.
4 Turn baby over onto his tummy (check that he is still warm).

Back Massage

Oil the baby's back.

1 Triangle effleurage
   Using as much of your hands as you can, start at baby's buttocks with your
   hands in a triangle shape, your thumb and fingers overlapping (Figure 11).
   Move very gently up baby's back, circle around both shoulders with each
   hand and return lightly down the sides of baby's body, back to his buttocks.
   Usually it is only possible to use your finger lengths on small babies, but as
   your baby gets bigger apply more of your hand. Repeat two to three times.

Opposite: Figures 11 & 12

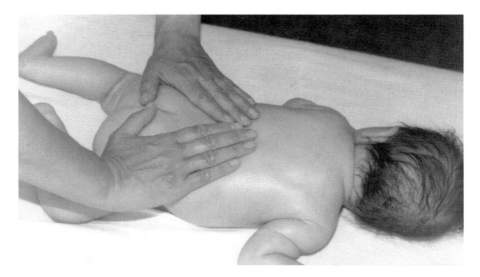

2 Thumb circles from buttocks to neck
   With your fingers underneath baby's hips, place each thumb on one of his
   buttocks, just above the top of his leg. Using slow, large, gentle circles, move
   your thumbs gradually up his back until you reach his shoulders (Figure 12).
   On reaching his shoulders, return your hands gently down the sides
   of his body. Repeat two to three times.
3 Repeat movement 1 two to three times.

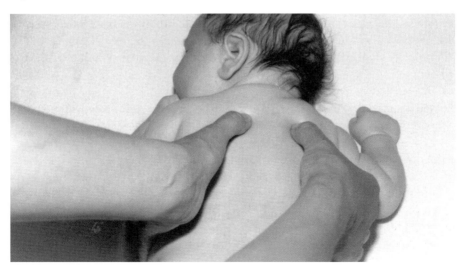

Backs of Legs and Feet

1 Repeat leg massage movements from 1 to 4 as described for the front of your
   baby's legs, but this time on the back of his legs.
   After completing this short massage on your baby, cover him up immediately
   with a soft warm towel (very important). Do not massage his face at this
   stage, as it is not always easy to avoid baby's eyes and mouth, especially
   when he is moving. When your baby is wrapped in the towel, pick him up
   and have a cuddle for a few minutes together. This increases the relaxation
   of the massage and is an ideal opportunity for you and your baby to spend
   relaxing moments together.

Case History

When my Penny's son Edward was only six weeks old he began to have a
'crabby' time between six and nine o'clock each night. This is very common
and is usually put down to 'infant colic'! Edward was breastfed and did not
appear to be in any pain; he simply did not want to settle.

It is at this time of day that a mother is tired after a busy day with her children –
and a father, having worked all day, is also ready to relax. Perhaps the baby can
sense this? Certainly, all of Penny's children could sense mealtimes, almost
waking up to order when it was time to eat! The home environment can affect a
child in very subtle ways, and Edward was probably expressing the deep
tiredness that ran throughout the whole household at this time. His sister,
Eleanor, who was nearly two, was also demanding in the early evening, but
fortunately slept well when put to bed – with her favourite smell of lavender,
of course!

It was decided to change Edward's bath and massage time from the morning,
when he was happy and relaxed, to six o'clock in the evening.

One drop of rose otto was used in his bath and, after several minutes of bath
play, he was wrapped in a warm towel. After a few minutes of cuddling, Penny
would massage his scalp, gently rotating her fingers over his head, stroking back
from the forehead to his nape.

Using a blend of rose otto (2 drops), frankincense (2 drops) and ylang ylang (1 drop) in 50 ml of grapeseed, she would then massage Edward's hands and feet. It was a wonderful opportunity to count and look at his tiny little toes and marvel at creation!

After the second treatment, Edward was already much calmer and more ready for his cot. After the third treatment, there were no problems with him at all.

The 'side-effect' was that Penny too was much calmer, having psyched herself up for half an hour of total dedication to him, rather than trying to carry on regardless and becoming irritated by his noise.

As he became older she began to do the massage with Edward lying in his cot, where he learned to fall asleep naturally.

Perhaps the greatest lesson learned, was that all children need is mum and her attention. Once they have been assured of that, they do become much more relaxed. We have followed this principle throughout our childrens' childhood, knowing that the more one says 'just a minute' or 'later', the more frustrated one becomes, as well as the children. If we mothers make time for play, homework and talk, then children are much happier to let us do our housework, etc. afterwards. A stitch in time, perhaps?

Massaging Older Children

When your baby is no longer a baby, but a toddler – and then a child – you will need to adapt the techniques, as suggested by the following massage. However, it may no longer be necessary to do a whole body massage, indeed, the older the child, the longer a full body massage will take. If you have more than one child you would spend most of your life doing massage! So we recommend that you do part massage, only using the whole massage perhaps once a week – or just on special occasions.

On a practical note, if you have never massaged your child before, the toddler stage is the hardest at which to begin. Toddlers have a very short attention span and simply walk away, leaving you with your lovely massage oil still on your hands! Start with very short massage sessions on the feet, then the hands, before attempting larger areas. The best time is just after a bath or, if you have time, first thing in the morning before the socks go on!

Back Massage

Back massage is very beneficial for stress, general relaxation, insomnia, aches and pains, shoulder tension and breathing difficulties. It will also help girls with Rett Syndrome (*see page 60*) to relax before a meal, helping the parents greatly with feeding.

Before starting the back massage, make sure your child is lying comfortably face down with perhaps a small pillow underneath his abdomen for support. The lower half of his body should be covered with a large soft towel and possibly a blanket, as heat is lost through the body during massage and your child will begin to feel cold if care is not taken. The best way to do this is to tuck the end of the towel into your child's pants (at buttock crease level), letting the rest of the towel fall down over his legs and covering them.

Take a very small amount of oil from your pre-mixed bottle (*see Chapter 4*) into the palm of one hand. Using both hands, rub your palms together gently until the oil is warmed. Place both hands just above the towel and lightly apply the oil all over your child's back in upward, circular movements. There should be enough oil to enable your hands to glide smoothly over his body; however, be careful not to apply too much, as it is not only difficult to massage well with too much oil, but a residue left on the skin will make your child feel uncomfortable and possibly stain his clothing.

Stand on the right side of your child (*see also page 126, point 6*).

1 Whole back effleurage
   Place both hands at the base of your child's spine, your thumbs touching and fingers pointing slightly towards each other and towards his head (Figure 13). Relax the whole of each hand and gently push them up to his shoulders, separating them around each shoulder and return gently to the base of his spine down each side of his body. Repeat five or six times.

Opposite: Figures 13 & 14

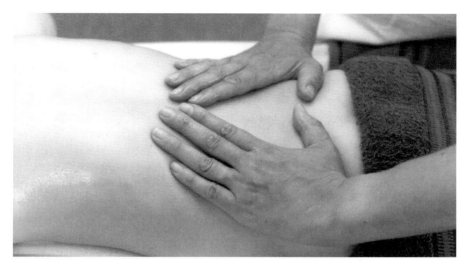

2 Thumb circling up spine

Place your thumbs on either side of your child's spine, just above the buttock crease. Supporting your hands by gently spreading your fingers towards the sides of his body, make slow circling movements (with your thumbs up) towards the nape of his neck (Figure 14). Take your hands across his shoulders and return to the base of his spine gently down the sides of his body with the whole hands of your hands. Repeat this thumb circling movement five or six times.

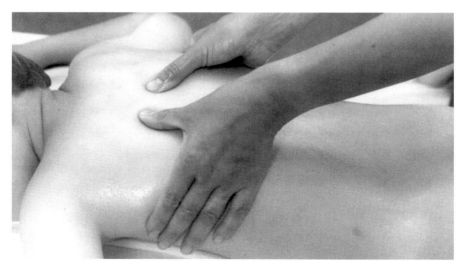

3 Alternate hand stroking

Starting on the left-hand side of your child's body with your left hand on his lower back (fingers facing the spine), slide your hand upwards, followed by your right hand on the same side (fingers facing the side of her body). Using short strokes with alternate hands, work up his back to his shoulder (Figure 15). Keeping one hand on his shoulder, start again at the bottom of his back and repeat the movement five or six times from base to shoulder. On the last movement, finish at your child's shoulder with your left hand and start on the right side (lower back) of his body with your right hand. Repeat on the right side five or six times, placing your left hand on his left shoulder for the last downward stroke, so that both hands finish at the base of his spine.

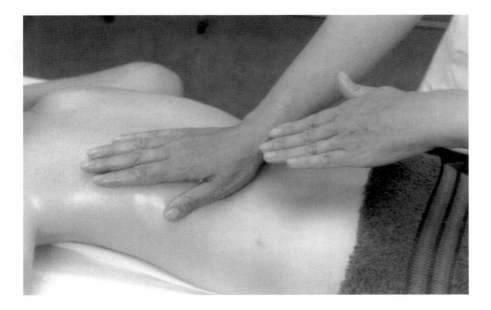

Figure 15

4 Zig-zag movements towards sides of body

Turn to face the side of your child's body, turning your hands so that your palms lie side by side on the base of his spine, your fingers pointing away to the left side of his back (Figure 16). Gently slide your left hand over to the left side of his body and your right hand to the right side of his body. Return both hands to his spine on a diagonal, so they are 10 – 12 cm (4 – 5 in) further up her spine and your right hand continues to the left side of his body, your left hand coming all the way to the right side. Repeat until both hands are at shoulder level and then return to the base of his spine by sliding each hand down the sides of his body lightly. Repeat five times, ending at his shoulders.

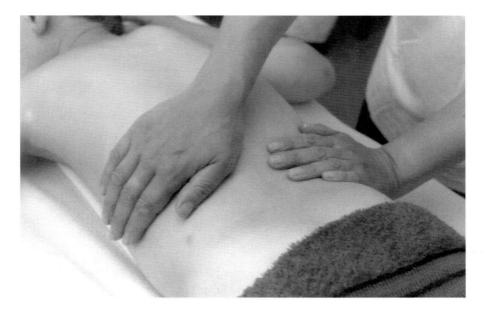

Figure 16

5 Butterfly circles round shoulder blades
   At shoulder level, place both hands side by side with your fingers pointing towards your child's head. Move them up to his neck, separate your hands and draw a circle with each hand at the same time around his shoulder blades, joining your hands together again on his spine (Figure 17). Repeat five or six times, finishing when each of your hands is on each of his shoulders.

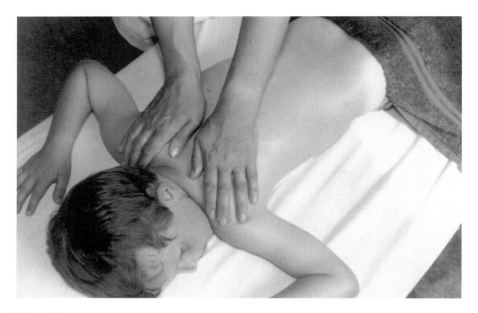

Figure 17

6 Thumb circles across shoulders
   Slide your fingers over your child's shoulder to the outer edge, leaving your
   thumbs at the top of his back. Making large circles with your thumbs, move
   towards his spine and out again to his shoulder (Figure 18). Repeat five or six
   times. Bring your hands gently down the sides of his body to the base
   of his spine.
7 Repeat movement 1.
8 Cover his back with a warm towel.

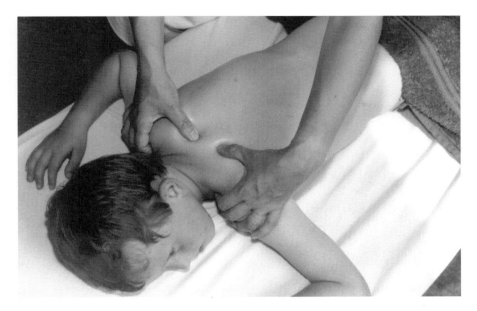

Figure 18

Leg Massage

Leg massage is beneficial for the following conditions: poor circulation, growing pains, hyperactivity, sports injuries, muscle fatigue, general stress and tension, all skin conditions. It is particularly good for girls with Rett Syndrome, where the legs are blue due to poor circulation (the pressure on the upward part of movement 1 (below) can be fairly strong to give such girls the greatest benefit).

Back of Legs

Apply oil to both of your child's legs. Cover his left leg with a towel – work up his right (nearest) leg first.

1 Whole leg effleurage
   Holding your child's right foot with your left hand, place the palm of your right hand on his ankle and allow your fingers to drape around his inner ankle (Figure 19). Sweep your whole hand up to the top of his thigh. Turn your hand towards his outer thigh and return gently down his outside leg to the ankle. Repeat five or six times.

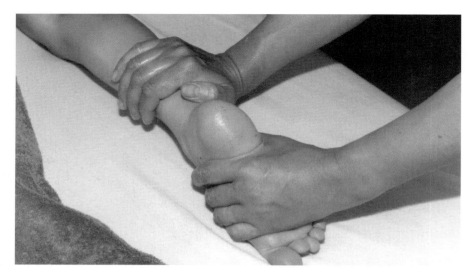

2 Effleurage to knee

Slide your right hand from your child's ankle to knee, holding it there until your left hand has moved from his foot to his ankle and also swept up to his knee (Figure 20). Using alternate hands, sweep from ankle to knee. Repeat five or six times, finishing with your left hand on his ankle and your right hand free.

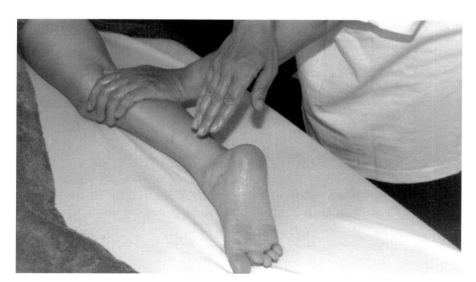

3 Circling up calf

Move round to face your child's feet (standing or kneeling at the bottom end of his body). Place both thumbs side by side on his ankle and make slow circling movements up his calf from the ankle to the knee, allowing your fingers to drape either side of his leg (Figure 21). On reaching the knee crease, separate your thumbs and return with your hands down each side of his leg to the ankle. Repeat five or six times, finishing the last movement at the knee crease.

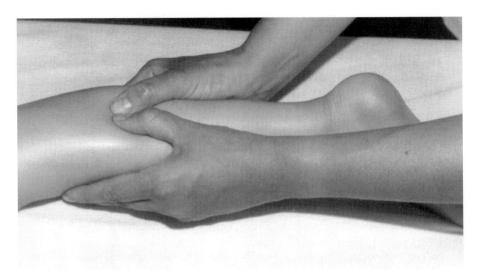

Figure 21

4 Inner thigh stroking

Move back round to the side of your child's body at knee level, without losing contact. Beginning with your left hand, place it just above knee level on his inner thigh. Draw your hand across his leg towards you, repeating the stroke with your right hand on his inner thigh before taking your left hand off (Figure 22). Move up his inner thigh to the top of his leg, progressing with each stroke and, on reaching the top with your right hand, start at his knee again with your left hand. Repeat five or six times.

Opposite: Figures 19 & 20

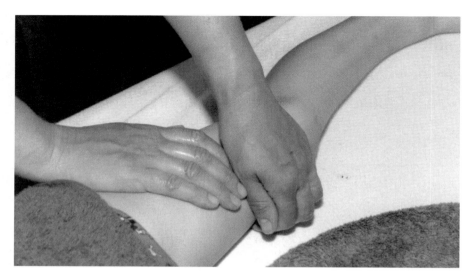

Figure 22

When your right hand has reached the top for the last time, bring it across the top of your child's leg, turning your hand to stroke down to his ankle.

5 Repeat movement 1 five or six times, finishing at the ankle
   A For the left leg, move round to the other side of your child's body and repeat the massage, reading left hand instead of right and right hand instead of left.
   B Cover his legs with a warm towel.

Front of Legs
Apply oil to both of your child's legs and cover up the leg furthest away from you. You are still working from the right-hand side of his body.

1 Whole leg effleurage
   Holding his right foot with your left hand, place the palm of your right hand on his ankle, allowing the fingers to drape around his inner ankle (Figure 23). Sweep your left hand up to the top of his thigh. Turn your hand towards his outer thigh and return gently down his outside leg to the ankle. Repeat five or six times.

Opposite: Figures 23 & 24

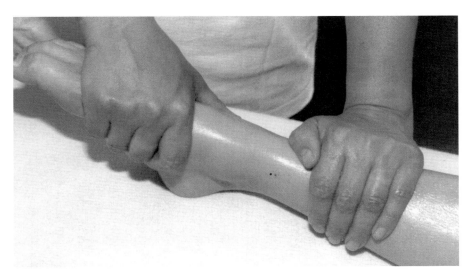

2 Effleurage to knee

Slide your right hand from ankle to knee, holding it there until your left
hand has moved from the foot to the ankle and also swept up to the knee.
Using alternate hands, sweep from ankle to knee (Figure 24). Repeat five or
six times, finishing with your left hand on your child's ankle and your right
hand free.

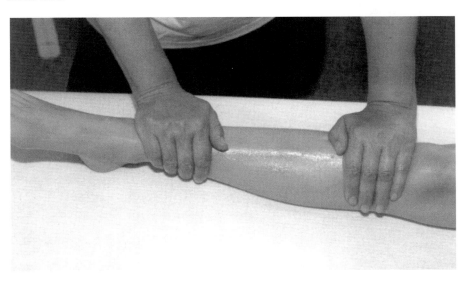

3 Thumb circles around knee cap
   With both thumbs under your child's knee cap, supported by your fingers, make small thumb circles under and around his knee cap, meeting at the top centre (Figure 25). Slide back to the starting position and repeat five or six times.

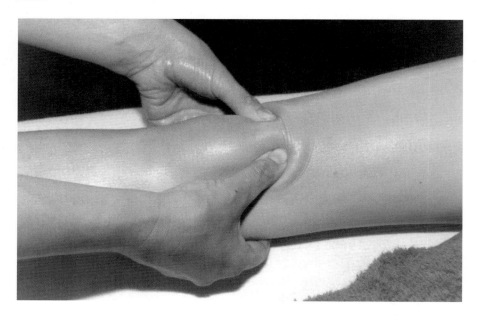

Figure 25

4 Inner thigh stroking
   Move back round to the side of your child at knee level, without losing contact. Beginning with your left hand, place it just above his knee on his inner thigh. Draw your hand across his leg towards you, starting again with your right hand on his inner thigh before taking your left hand off (Figure 26). Move up his inner thigh to the top of his leg, progressing with each stroke. On reaching the top with your right hand, start at the knee again with your left hand. Repeat five or six times.

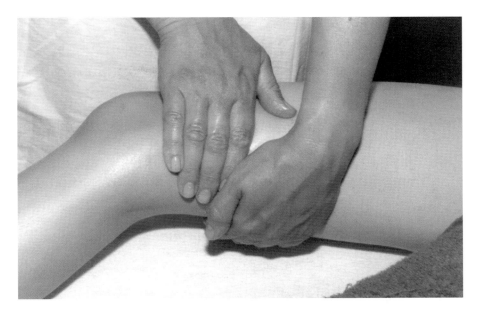

Figure 26

When your right hand has reached the top for the last time, bring it across the top of her leg, turning your hand to stroke down to his ankle.

5 Repeat movement 1 five or six times.
   A To massage your child's left leg, move round to other side of his body and repeat the massage as described above, reading left hand instead of right and right hand instead of left.
   B Cover his legs with a warm towel.

Foot Massage

Foot massage is beneficial for the following: poor circulation, cold feet, skin conditions, cramp, fungal infections.

1 Foot rotation
   Holding the top of your child's foot with one hand, and his ankle with the other, circle his foot gently three times clockwise and three times anticlockwise (Figure 27).

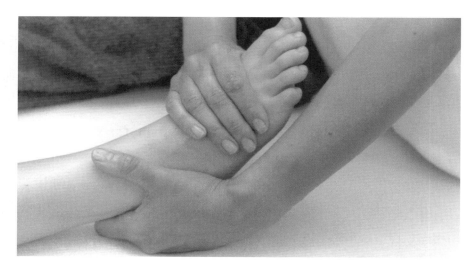

2 Effleurage
   Place one hand behind the other, both sets of fingers pointing in opposite
   directions, at the top of your child's foot (that is, on his toes). Move both
   hands up his foot to the ankle. Leaving one hand on his ankle, slide the other
   hand to the sole of his foot and pull both hands up to his toes, squeezing as
   you go (Figures 28 and 29). Repeat five or six times.

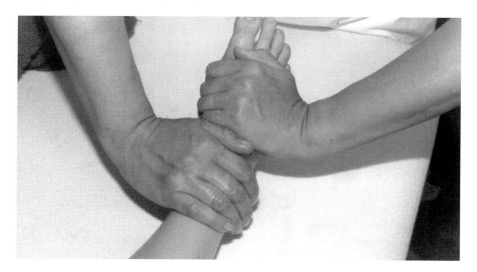

Above: Figures 27 & 28

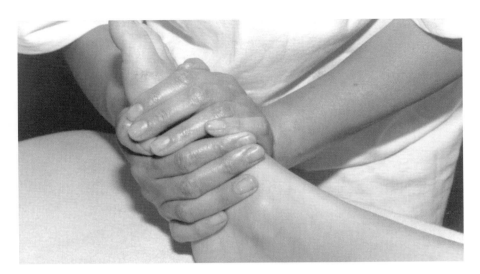

3 Friction circles on top of foot
   Starting at your child's toes, using both thumbs and holding the underside of
   his foot with your fingers, make small thumb circles between toes 1 and 2,
   then 3 and 4, working down to the arch of the foot (Figure 30). Gently slide
   back and repeat between toes 2 and 3, then 4 and 5. Do each channel twice.

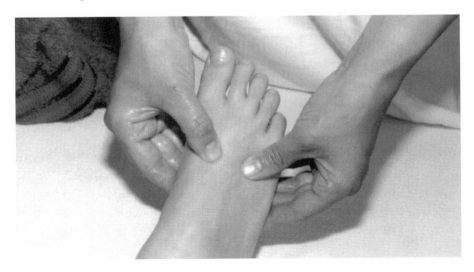

Above: Figures 29 & 30

4 Sole circles
   Hold your child's foot in one hand and with the thumb of the other hand,
   circle gently on the soft part of his sole, under the ball of his foot
   (Figure 31).

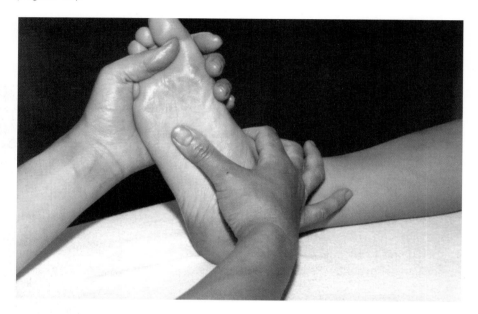

Figure 31

5 Repeat movement 2 five or six times

Abdomen Massage

Abdomen massage is useful for the following: anxiety, constipation, diarrhoea,
enteritis, flatulence, indigestion, colic and nausea.

N.B. Because the tissues of the abdomen have no skeletal support, pressure
must be very gentle and the whole hand used where possible.

Stand at the right hand side of your child's body.

Opposite: Figures 32 and 33

1 Diamond effleurage

Place both hands with fingertips at the base of your child's breastbone and, from here, spread your hands, one underneath each side of his rib cage, to the waist. Turn your hands, wrapping your fingers underneath your child's waist, and then draw your hands towards each other, meeting just below his navel (Figures 32 and 33). Slide both hands up to his breastbone and repeat the movement five or six times. Finish the last movement underneath his navel.

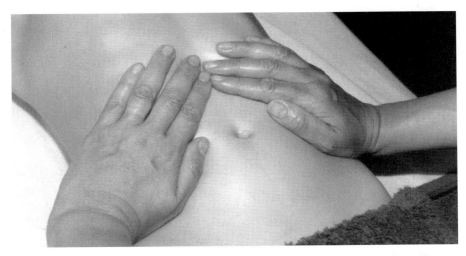

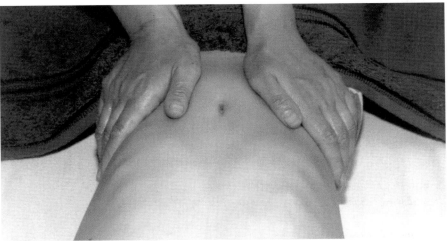

2 Circular movement
Leaving one hand on your child's breastbone, move the other slowly in a
large circle around his navel in a clockwise direction (Figure 34). Repeat five
or six times.

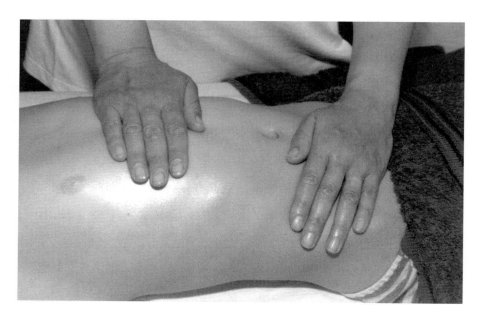

Figure 34

3 Side stroking
Start this movement when your circling hand reaches the hip furthest away
from you (left). Take your hand to the side of your child's body and gently
pull your hand upwards towards you, repeating the same lifting stroke
slightly higher up her body with the other hand (Figure 35). Use this
alternate hand-stroking movement until reaching the chest. Begin again at his
hip and repeat five or six times. After completing the last movement keep one
hand on that side of his body and, while moving round to the other side of
your child's body, turn and slide your hand over and down to his right hip
and begin the movement on that side of her body. Repeat five or six times,
finishing at chest level.

Opposite: *Figures 35 & 36*

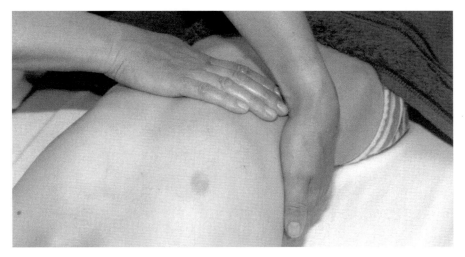

4 Upward stroking
   Leaving one hand on the side of his body, place the other hand across his
   abdomen below the navel (Figure 36). Slide your whole hand up the centre of
   his abdomen to the breastbone. Move the other hand to below his navel to
   repeat the same movement. Using alternate hands, complete five or six
   upward stroking movements, finishing at the breastbone.
5 Repeat movement number 1.
   Cover him with a warm towel.

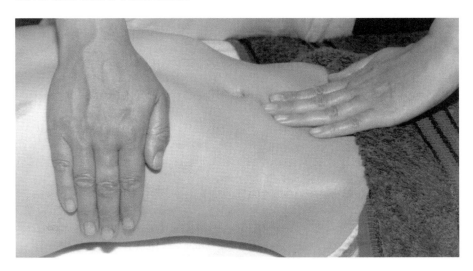

Arm Massage

Arm massage is useful for the following: aches and pains, skin conditions, cramp and tension.

1 Effleurage
   Hold your child's right hand with your left hand and move your right hand gently up her arm to his shoulder; turn and return to his wrist (Figure 37). Repeat five or six times.

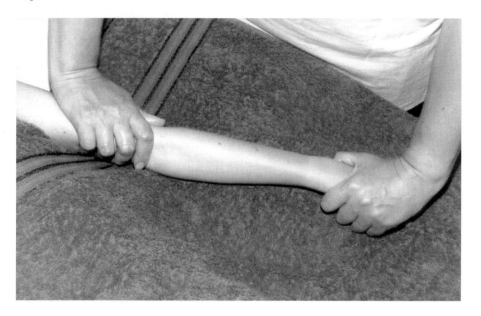

Figure 37

2 Half-way effleurage
   Repeat movement number 1 up to your child's elbow and return to his wrist five or six times.
3 Inner arm zig-zag
   Place both thumbs on your child's inside wrist just below his palm. Slide your thumbs past each other and back again in a zig zag movement across his wrist (Figure 38). Move up his inner arm in the same manner up to his elbow crease and return gently to his wrist. Repeat five or six times.

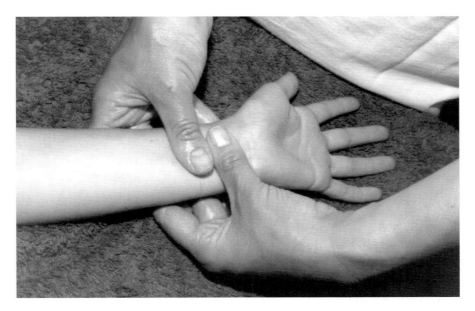

Figure 38

4 Repeat movement number 1.

 A Repeat on your child's right arm, remembering to change 'left' to 'right' when following the movements described above.

Hand Massage

Hand massage is beneficial for the following: cramp, poor circulation, muscle fatigue, poor nail growth, skin conditions, general relaxation, hyperactivity.

1 Wrist rotation
 Holding your child's wrist steady with one hand, hold his fingers in your other hand. Move his hand in three clockwise circles and then three anticlockwise circles (Figure 39).

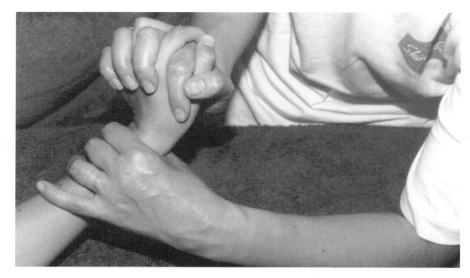

2 Circle frictions on back of hand
   Holding his hand, place your thumbs so that one is between his 2nd and 3rd
   fingers, the other between his 4th and 5th fingers. Move between the tendons
   towards the wrist in small circular movements (Figure 40). Move the thumbs
   to between thumb and 2nd finger, and 3rd and 4th finger and repeat the
   movement down these two channels three times.

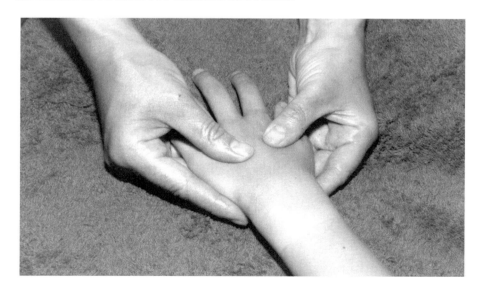

3 Finger massage
   With one of your hands, hold your child's hand, using the other hand to
   massage each finger in turn by moving from the base of each finger to the tip
   in small circles with your thumb (Figure 41).

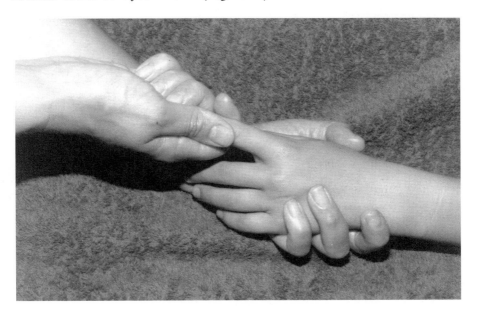

Figure 41

4 Palm circling
   Turn your child's hand over and, holding it with one hand, use the thumb
   of your other hand to move in slow circles around the centre of his palm
   (Figure 42).

***Opposite:** Figures 39 & 40*

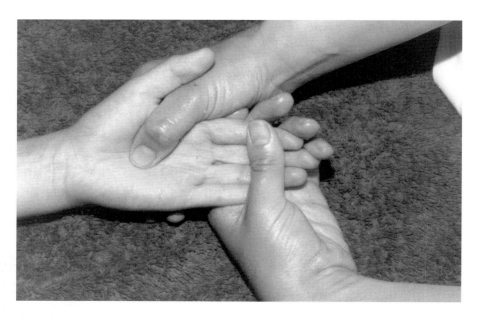

5 Hand holding
   To finish the massage, hold your child's hand in both of yours (like a sandwich) for at least 30 seconds before letting go (Figure 43).

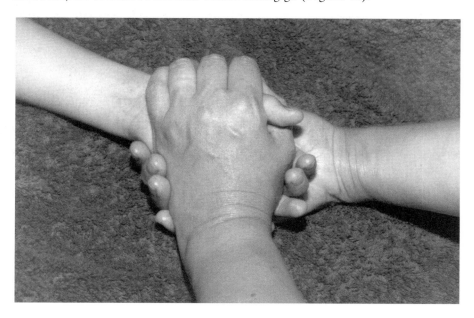

Chest and Neck Massage

Chest and neck massage is useful for the following: coughs, colds, catarrh, bronchitis, asthma, anxiety, heartburn, neck and shoulder tension.

Leave your child covered warmly up to her armpits and position yourself behind his head.

1 Chest effleurage
  Place both hands on his upper chest (Figure 44). Sweep your hands out to his armpits and round his shoulders, turning them to continue the movement under her shoulder to the back of his neck (Figure 45). Repeat five or six times.

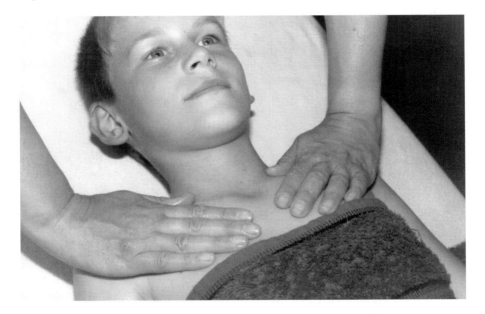

Figure 44

Opposite: Figures 42 & 43

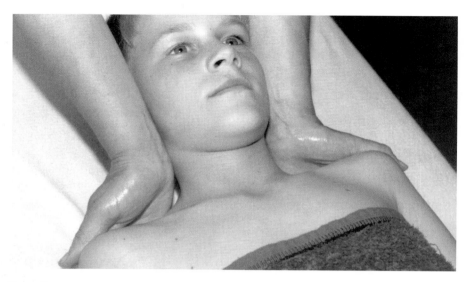

2 Kneading

Place your fingers under her shoulders with your thumbs on top. Rotating your fingers and thumbs, work in towards his neck (Figure 46). Slide gently back to his shoulder points and repeat five or six times.

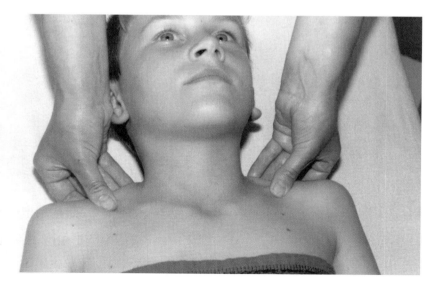

Above: Figures 45 & 46

3 Upward neck stroking
   Starting at the right side of his neck, use the fingers of alternate hands to
   stroke from collar bone to jaw, working over to the left side and back again
   (Figure 47). Repeat three times.
4 Repeat movement number 1.

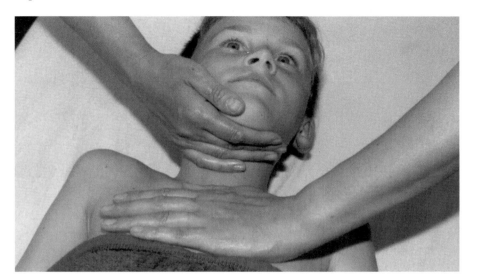

Figure 47

Face Massage

Face massage is difficult to do on a young child who cannot keep still. There is
always a need to be careful to avoid getting oil in your child's eyes or mouth, so
choose your moments carefully – such as when she is over five years old!

Face massage is beneficial for the following: headache, sinus, skin problems,
tension and toothache.

1 Jaw cupping
   Cup the right side of your child's jaw with your left hand and sweep over to
   the left side of her jaw (Figure 48). Place your right hand on the left side of
   her jaw and sweep to the right side. Continue to alternate the hands like this
   for five or six movements.

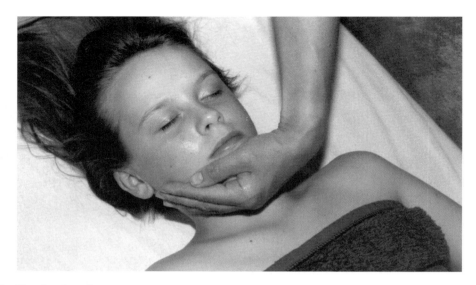

2 Cheek triangles
  Using the index, middle and ring fingers of both hands, start at the corners of
  your child's mouth, then move up each side of her nose and slide under her
  eyes to her temples (Figure 49). Gently return down the outside of her
  cheeks and along her jaw back to her mouth. Repeat five or six times. Finish
  by sliding up each side of her nose onto her forehead.

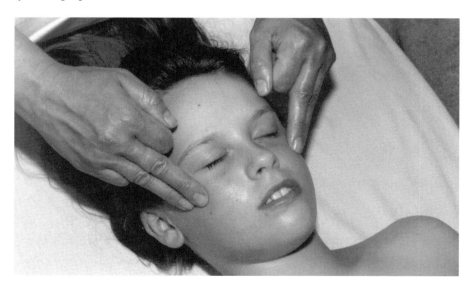

3 Forehead stroking
Using the finger lengths of alternating hands, move from your child's brow to her hairline five or six times (Figure 50).

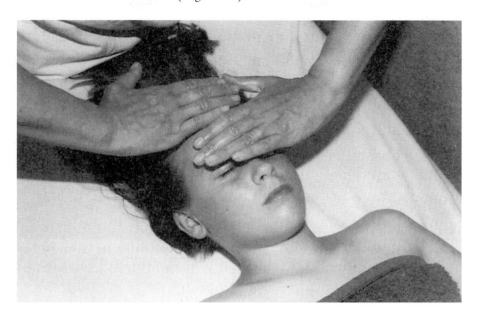

Figure 50

4 Eye circling
Using the ring and middle fingers of each hand, stroke from your child's centre brow along brow line and circle gently past her temples and under each eye (Figures 51 and 52, overleaf). Repeat five or six times, finishing the massage by gently resting your fingers on her temples for a few seconds.

Opposite: Figures 48 & 49

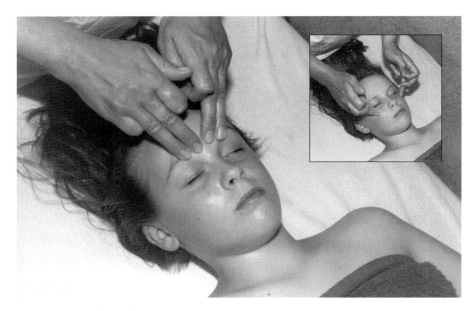

Above: Figures 51 & 52

Scalp Massage

Scalp massage is beneficial for the following: slow hair growth, fine hair, dandruff, psoriasis, eczema, dull lifeless hair, headaches, examination stress, insomnia and tension.

Scalp massage can be done with or without oil, depending on the treatment being given. Scalp tonic is also suitable where the hair is lifeless, dull or otherwise in poor condition.

N.B. Initially, scalp massage can loosen hair ready to fall out, giving the appearance of excessive hair loss. This loss is less apparent after only one day and disappears with regular scalp massage, which can actually help prevent hair loss.

1 Scalp stroking
   Using the fingers of each hand, alternately 'rake' gently through your child's hair from her facial outline to her crown (Figure 53).

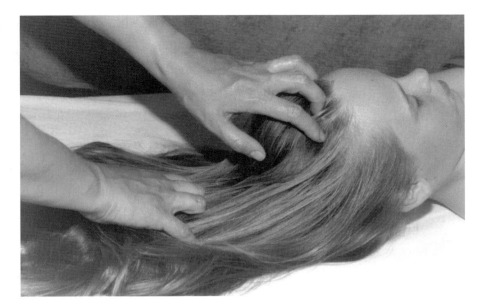

Figure 53

2 Scalp frictions
   Gently place the pads of your fingers on your child's scalp and move her skin
   over the bone underneath (Figure 54, overleaf). After a few seconds, move to
   a new area and repeat. Move and repeat again until her whole head has been
   covered.
3 Repeat movement number 1.

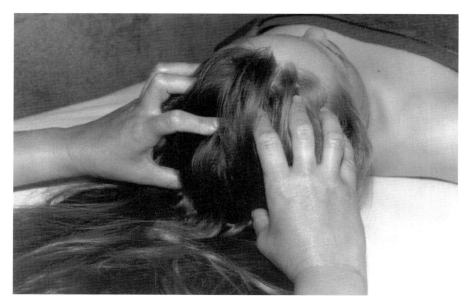

Figure 54

Case Histories

Sam's mother, Jane, had been told that Sam had high energy levels – he was mildly hyperactive. She had already tried to massage Sam, who was 3, but had had difficulty in catching him and making him stay still for long enough to receive the massage. Jane had also spoken to a dietitian and changed Sam's diet accordingly, omitting highly coloured, high-energy foods (such as cola, orange and other drinks high in additives – and very brightly coloured sweets).

We recommended that Jane use sandalwood in a vaporizer and play a relaxation music tape for half an hour before approaching Sam with massage oil. The massage oil contained 10 ml hypericum, 40 ml sunflower, 3 drops sandalwood, 3 drops ylang ylang and 2 drops lavender.

For the first 'treatment' we suggested Jane try to massage only one of Sam's hands at first. For this Sam could manage to sit still. Jane continued to massage alternate hands for six consecutive days. On the seventh day she attempted to massage both hands, but Sam did not want to sit still for this length of time.

After 10 days, however, Sam did allow Jane to massage both hands. By the sixteenth day, Sam was having both hands *and* arms massaged. Jane told me on the phone that as soon as she switched on her vaporizer and tape recorder, Sam came over to her for his massage, so he obviously enjoyed it!

Jane very patiently added to the massage slowly over a period of eight weeks, eventually building up to a full massage. The change in Sam when we saw him after this time was incredible. Still a very talkative, lively and enthusiastic 3-year-old, he was no longer bored, aggressive or fidgety.

Jane began to alternate the massage with oils in the bath, and has been very impressed by the effect of the oils on Sam – and herself!

Hannah was 12 years old when she came to our clinic with exam nerves. She was a talented young pianist and had an important piano exam to sit. Shirley gave her a chest, face and scalp massage using 1 drop each of rosemary, rosewood and sweet thyme in 10 ml of grapeseed (this mixture lasted for three treatments) to relax and uplift her.

The massage relieved the tension in her neck and shoulders, and she told Shirley that the smell had 'strengthened' her. After her three treatments, given at three-day intervals, Hannah took her exam without fear and passed. She has said she will continue treatment for future GCSE exams in the hope that she will have similar success!

Jennifer (aged 8) suffers with Rett Syndrome (*see page 60*). Jennifer's circulation was such that her lower legs were bluish-purple and her mother, Anne, was having difficulty feeding her because of her hands 'flailing' continuously around her face (one of the symptoms of Rett Syndrome).

Anne came to Shirley for advice, following a lecture on aromatherapy which Shirley had given at the Rett Syndrome Society AGM. She massaged Jennifer's back and legs and after a few minutes Jennifer began to smile at her mother (at first she was not sure what was happening). The leg massage (using upward strokes only) was to help Jennifer's circulation; the back massage was to relax her as well as to help her circulation.

The oils Shirley used and gave Anne for Jennifer's legs were those which stimulated the circulation, containing benzoin, black pepper, juniper and rosemary. she gave her pure oils in a little dropper bottle to use in Jennifer's bath – and the same oils diluted in hazelnut oil with a little calendula for massaging her legs. The oil used on Jennifer's back was a mix for stress, containing basil, juniper, lavender and sandalwood. Shirley taught Jennifer's mother how to give a simple massage to her daughter's legs and back, giving her the relaxing oils she would need.

After less than a week, a delighted Anne telephoned Shirley to say that the back massage so relaxed Jennifer that she kept her hands still throughout every meal, which had reduced the stress Anne normally felt while feeding her.

Anne returned after two weeks for a professional treatment for Jennifer – and another lesson. Jennifer's legs were already a healthier colour, which greatly pleased me, as well as her mother! Anne is continuing to give Jennifer the regular massage treatments to maintain the benefits gained.

Conclusion

Massage is a therapy in its own right, and is exceedingly beneficial physically and mentally. However, when combined with the therapeutic, balancing effects of essential oils, we can far exceed the benefits of massage alone. The combined smells and the aroma/emotion reaction, the touch of the massage and the gentle stimulating effect of the essential oils on the body's healing mechanisms can produce results that will delight both you and your family.

7

Directory of Oils, Carriers and Methods of Use

Abdominal Pain
chamomile (Roman), ginger, lavender, mandarin, marjoram (sweet), sandalwood
hypericum, sunflower, water, white lotion
application, bath, compress, massage

Abscesses
See **Boils**

Aches & Pains (General)
eucalyptus (*smithii*), frankincense, ginger, lavender, marjoram, rosemary
water, hypericum, sunflower
application, bath, compress, massage

Acne
geranium, lavender, rosewood, sandalwood, tea tree, thyme (sweet)
hazelnut, water, white lotion
application, bath, facial splash, massage

Air Antiseptic
lemon
air
inhalation, vaporization

Allergies
bergamot, chamomile (Roman), geranium*, lavender
calendula, cream, grapeseed, sunflower, water, white lotion
application, bath, massage

Anger
chamomile (Roman)
air, water
bath, inhalation, vaporization

Anxiety
chamomile (Roman), geranium, lavender, mandarin, marjoram (sweet), orange
    (sweet), rose otto, rosewood, sandalwood, tea tree, thyme (sweet), ylang ylang
lime blossom, sunflower, water, white lotion
bath, inhalation, massage, vaporization

Agitation
bergamot, rosewood
air
application

Appetite Loss
bergamot, chamomile (Roman), lemon, mandarin
air, water, sunflower, sweet almond, white lotion
application, bath, inhalation, massage (abdomen), vaporization

Arthritis/Rheumatism
eucalyptus (*smithii*), lavender, marjoram (sweet), rosemary
carrot, hypericum, lime blossom, sunflower
water
bath, massage

Asthma
chamomile (Roman), eucalyptus (*smithii*), frankincense, lavender, mandarin,
    marjoram (sweet), rose otto, thyme (sweet)
air, cream, sunflower, white lotion
application, massage, vaporization

Athlete's Foot
geranium, lavender, tea tree
calendula, cream, grapeseed, water, white lotion
application, footbath, massage

Bad Breath
thyme (sweet)
water
gargle, mouth wash

Bedwetting
cypress, marjoram (sweet)*, rosemary
hypericum, water
bath, massage (abdomen)

Blisters
cedarwood, cypress, geranium, lavender
calendula, hypericum, rose hip, sunflower, water, white lotion
application, compress

Boils
chamomile (Roman), lemon, rosewood, tea tree
calendula, hypericum, rose hip, white lotion
application

Broken Capillaries
See **Thread veins**

Bronchitis
cedarwood, cypress, eucalyptus (*smithii*), frankincense, lavender, marjoram
   (sweet), rosemary, rose otto, rosewood, sandalwood, tea tree, thyme (sweet)
air, hypericum, sunflower, water, white lotion
bath, chest massage, vaporization

Bruises
cypress, eucalyptus (*smithii*), lavender, lemon, rosemary
calendula, hypericum, olive, water, white lotion
application, compress

Burns (Minor)
chamomile (Roman), frankincense, lavender, rosemary, rose otto
carrot, hypericum, olive, rose hip, water, white lotion
application, bath, compress

Catarrh
See **Common cold**

Chest Infection
See **Bronchitis**

Chicken Pox
chamomile (Roman)*, frankincense*, geranium*, lavender, lemon*, rose otto
carrot, sweet almond, water, white lotion
application, bath, massage

Chilblains
chamomile (Roman), cypress, lavender, lemon, sandalwood*
calendula, carrot, sunflower, water, white lotion
application, bath (hand/foot)

Circulation Problems
bergamot
water
bath

Tonic/Sluggish/Cold Feet cedarwood, eucalyptus (*smithii*), geranium, ginger,
    lavender, lemon, marjoram (sweet), rosemary, rose otto
avocado, calendula, sunflower, white lotion
application, massage

Cold Sores
bergamot, eucalyptus (*smithii*), geranium, lavender
hypericum, water, white lotion
application, bath

Colic
bergamot, chamomile (Roman), ginger, mandarin, marjoram (sweet), rosemary,
    ylang ylang
calendula, grapeseed, water, white lotion
application, bath, massage, weak (chamomile) tea
See also **Nausea**

Common Cold
cedarwood, eucalyptus (*smithii*), lemon, rosemary, rose otto, sandalwood,
    tea tree, thyme (sweet)
air, carrot, grapeseed sunflower, water, white lotion
application, bath, massage, vaporization

Constipation
ginger, mandarin, orange (sweet), rosemary
avocado, sunflower, water
application, bath, massage (abdomen)

Coughs
cedarwood, eucalyptus (*smithii*), marjoram (sweet), rosemary, sandalwood,
    thyme (sweet)
air, hypericum, sunflower, white lotion
chest massage, vaporization

Spasmodic lavender

Whooping cypress, marjoram (sweet)

Cradle Cap
cedarwood, lavender, rosemary, sandalwood
olive, sweet almond
scalp massage

Cramp
See **Muscles**

Croup
eucalyptus (*smithii*), marjoram (sweet), rosewood, sandalwood, thyme (sweet)
white lotion
application, inhalation, vaporization

Crying (Distress)
chamomile (Roman), cypress, frankincense, geranium, lavender, rose otto,
   ylang ylang
air, lime blossom, water
bath, inhalation, massage, vaporization

Cuts
bergamot, chamomile (Roman), geranium, lavender, rosemary, rose otto,
   tea tree
calendula, hypericum, rose hip, water, white lotion
application, bath

Cystitis
cedarwood, eucalyptus (*smithii*), sandalwood, thyme (sweet)
water
bath

Dandruff
cedarwood, geranium*, lemon, rosemary, tea tree
grapeseed, olive, sweet almond, water
hair rinse, massage, scalp tonic

Day-dreaming
marjoram (sweet)
air
bath, inhalation, vaporization

Dermatitis
See Eczema and Nappy Rash

Depression
bergamot, chamomile (Roman), frankincense, geranium, orange (sweet),
   rose otto, rosewood, sandalwood, tea tree
air, lime blossom, sunflower, water
bath, massage, vaporization

Diabetes
lemon, geranium, ylang ylang
sunflower, water, white lotion
application, bath, massage

Diarrhoea
chamomile (Roman), geranium, ginger, lemon, marjoram (sweet), sandalwood
calendula, sunflower, white lotion
application, massage

Distress
See **Crying**

Dry, Dull, Brittle Lifeless Hair
cedarwood, rosemary, ylang ylang
grapeseed, water
massage, scalp tonic
Also see Chapter 2

Dry Skin
rosewood, sandalwood
calendula, sweet almond, wheatgerm, white lotion
application

Earache
chamomile (Roman), lavender, tea tree, thyme (sweet)
hypericum, sweet almond, white lotion
massage

Eczema
bergamot, cedarwood, chamomile (Roman), frankincense*, geranium, lavender,
    rose otto, sandalwood, thyme
avocado, calendula, carrot, rose hip, sweet almond, water, white lotion
application, bath, massage

Epilepsy
See Chapter 5

Fever
See **High temperature**

Flatulence (wind)
chamomile (Roman), ginger, marjoram (sweet), rosemary
grapeseed, sunflower, sweet almond, white lotion
application, massage

Fluid retention
geranium, thyme (sweet)
avocado, grapeseed, sunflower, white lotion
massage (upwards)

Gastro-enteritis
ginger, mandarin*, marjoram (sweet)
air, calendula, sunflower, white lotion
application, massage (abdomen), vaporization
See also **Diarrhoea**

Greasy skin
lemon, ylang ylang
hazelnut, water, white lotion
application, facial splash

Grief
frankincense, rose otto
air, lime blossom, water
bath, inhalation, massage, vaporization

Gum infections and Gingivitis (inflammation)
tea tree, thyme (sweet), sweet almond
water
mouth wash

Hair and scalp
See Chapter 2 and **Dandruff, Dry, dull, brittle lifeless hair, Lice & nits**

Haemorrhoids
cypress, rose otto, tea tree
water, white lotion
application, bath

Hayfever
eucalyptus (*smithii*)*, grapeseed, rosewood*
air, water, white lotion
application, bath, inhalation, vaporization

Headaches (migraine)
chamomile (Roman), lavender, lemon
air, water
bath, inhalation

Heartburn
mandarin, marjoram (sweet), rosemary, sandalwood
white lotion
application

Hiccoughs
mandarin
air
inhalation

High temperature
eucalyptus (*smithii*)*
water
bath (tepid)

Hormonal imbalance (teenagers)
chamomile (Roman)*
lime blossom massage, water, white lotion
application, bath

Hyperactivity

bergamot, chamomile (Roman), frankincense, geranium, lavender, mandarin, marjoram (sweet), rose otto, sandalwood, thyme (sweet), ylang ylang
air, lime blossom, sunflower, water
bath, massage, vaporization

Hysteria

cypress
air
inhalation

Immune system

frankincense, lemon, rosewood*, tea tree, thyme
air, calendula, sunflower, water
bath, inhalation, massage

Impetigo

geranium, rosewood*, tea tree
calendula, carrot, hypericum, water, white lotion
application, bath, massage

Indigestion

See **Colic, Nausea, Sluggish digestion**

Inflammation

chamomile (Roman), lavender, rose otto
calendula, carrot, white lotion
application

Influenza

cypress, lemon
air, water
bath, inhalation, vaporization

Insect bites

chamomile (Roman), lavender, lemon, sandalwood, tea tree
carrot, olive, white lotion
application

Insect repellent
geranium
white lotion
application, spray

Insecurity
See **Depression**

Insomnia
bergamot, chamomile (Roman), lavender, lemon, mandarin, marjoram (sweet),
    sandalwood, ylang ylang
air, lime blossom, water, white lotion
application, bath, inhalation, massage

Invigorating (uplifting)
lemon, rosemary
air, water
bath, inhalation, vaporization

Irritability
chamomile (Roman), cypress
air, lime blossom
inhalation, massage, vaporization

Jaundice
geranium, lemon, mandarin, rosemary
white lotion
application

Kidney infections
eucalyptus (*smithii*)*, sandalwood
water, white lotion
application (small of the back), bath

Kidney tonic
frankincense*
water, white lotion
application, bath

Lice & Nits
eucalyptus (*smithii*)*, rosemary, tea tree, thyme (sweet)*
water
hair rinse

Liver tonic
lemon, mandarin, rosemary
avocado, calendula, sunflower, water
bath, massage

Measles
geranium, lavender, lemon*
carrot, water, white lotion
application, bath
Also see oils listed for **Cramp** *and* **High Temperature**

Moodiness
mandarin
air, bath, water
inhalation, vaporization

Mouth ulcers
bergamot, geranium, orange (sweet), rose otto
water
mouth wash

Muscles
Cramp
cypress*, eucalyptus (*smithii*)*, ginger, lavender, marjoram (sweet), rosemary
avocado, hypericum, lime blossom, sunflower, water, white lotion
application, bath, compress (hot/cold), massage

Injury
cypress, eucalyptus (*smithii*), ginger, lavender, marjoram (sweet)
carrot, hypericum, lime blossom (stress), water, white lotion

Tension
rose otto, rosewood
See also **Aches & Pains**

Nappy rash (contact dermatitis)
bergamot, chamomile (Roman), frankincense, geranium, lavender, rose otto,
  sandalwood
calendula, carrot, sunflower, water, white lotion
application, bath, massage
See also **Eczema** and **Thrush**

Nausea
bergamot, ginger, lemon, mandarin, orange (sweet), rosewood*
sunflower, sweet almond, white lotion
application, massage (abdomen and chest)

Nightmares
lemon, ylang ylang
air, lime blossom, water, white lotion
application, bath, inhalation, massage, vaporization

Nosebleeds
cypress, lemon
water
compress

Pimples
See **Acne** and **Greasy skin**

Psoriasis
bergamot, chamomile (Roman), lavender
calendula, carrot, sweet almond, water, wheatgerm
bath, massage

Rashes
chamomile (Roman), lavender, rose otto, sandalwood
calendula, carrot, water, white lotion
application, bath

Ringworm
geranium, rose otto*, tea tree, thyme (sweet)
water, white lotion
application, bath

Scabies
chamomile (Roman), rosewood, tea tree, thyme (sweet)
water, white lotion
application, bath

Scar tissue
frankincense, geranium, lavender, rose otto
carrot, rose hip, white lotion
application

Shingles
See Chicken pox

Sinus trouble
See Common cold

Skin conditions
See Acne, Dry skin, Eczema, Greasy skin, Impetigo, Psoriasis,
   Scabies and Rashes

Sore throat
See Coughs

Spots
See Acne

Stress
See Anxiety

Sunburn
chamomile (Roman), lavender, rose otto, sandalwood
carrot, rose hip, water, white lotion
application, bath

Sluggish digestion
lemon, orange (sweet)
calendula, sunflower, water, white lotion
application (facial), bath, massage

Teething (toothache)
chamomile (Roman), ginger, lavender, marjoram (sweet), tea tree
hypericum, white lotion
application

Temper tantrums
lavender, mandarin, rose otto, sandalwood, ylang ylang
air, lime blossom, sunflower, water
bath, inhalation, massage

Thread veins
cypress, lemon
calendula, white lotion
application

Threadworms (roundworms)
chamomile (Roman) (itchiness), eucalyptus (*smithii*)*, lavender (itchiness),
    tea tree, thyme (sweet)
water, white lotion
application (hand and anal), bath

Throat infections
lavender, sandalwood, tea tree, thyme (sweet)
water, white lotion
application, gargle (if able)

Thrush
geranium, lavender, lemon, rosewood, tea tree, thyme (sweet)
calendula, sunflower, water, white lotion (nappy rash)
application, bath, massage

Timidity
ginger
air, grapeseed
inhalation, massage, vaporization

Tonsillitis
See **Throat infections**

Travel sickness
bergamot, chamomile (Roman)*, ginger, lavender, lemon, orange (sweet),
    rosewood, sandalwood
air, white lotion
application (abdomen – prior to journey), inhalation

Ulcers
bergamot, thyme (sweet)
water, white lotion
application, compress

Urinary infections
sandalwood, tea tree, thyme (sweet)
white lotion
application

Verrucae
bergamot, geranium*, lemon, thyme (sweet)
water, white lotion
bath (foot), massage (foot)

Vomiting
See **Travel sickness**

Warts
See **Verrucae**

Wind
See **Flatulence**

Whooping cough
cypress, marjoram (sweet)
air, water, white lotion
application (throat and chest), inhalation, vaporization

Wounds
See **Burns** and **Cuts**

References

1992 *A – Z of Childhood Ailments*. Bounty Press
1994 *Family Medical Encyclopaedia: An illustrated guide*. Guild Publishing
Anckett A 1979 'Baby Massage – Alternative to drugs'. *Australian Nursing Journal* 9 (5)
Bennett G 1992 *Handbook of Clinical Dietetics*. Riverhead, Stratford–upon–Avon
Lawless J 1992 *The Encyclopaedia of Essential Oils*. Element, Shaftesbury
Mabey R 1988 *The Complete New Herbal*. Gaia Books Ltd, London
Price L 1995 *Alpha – Omega Essential Oils*.
Price L 1990 *Carrier Oils for Aromatherapy and Massage*. Riverhead, Stratford–upon–Avon
Price S 1995 *Aromatherapy for Health Professionals*. Churchill Livingstone, Edinburgh
Price S 1993 *Aromatherapy Workbook*. Thorsons, London
Ryman D 1984 *The Aromatherapy Handbook*. Daniels, Saffron Walden
Wingate P 1972 *The Penguin Medical Encyclopaedia*. Penguin

Bibliography

1978 *Reader's Digest Mothercare Book*. Reader's Digest
Franchomme P and Pénoël 1990 *Aromathérapie Exactement*. Jollois, Limoges
Kusmerick J 1992 *Aromatherapy for the Family*. The Institute of Classical Aromatherapy, Wigmore Publications
Price P 2003 *Aromatherapy and the Pregnant Woman*. Monograph, Penny Price Academy of Aromatherapy, Hinckley
Price L 1995 *Alpha – Omega Essential Oils*.
Price S 1991 *Aromatherapy for Common Ailments*. Gaia Books Ltd, London
Price L & S 1999 *Aromatherapy for Health Professionals*. Churchill Livingstone, Edinburgh

Useful Addresses

Products and Training

Penny Price Aromatherapy Ltd
The Stables
41 Leicester Road
Hinckley
Leics LE10 1LW
Tel: 01455 251020
Email: info@penny–price.com

**Sandra Day School of
    Health Studies**
185a Drake Street,
Rochdale,
OL11 1EF
Tel 01706 750302
Fax 01706750304
info@sandraday.com

Tilia Ltd,
418–1–1–1, K–Royal Hotel, E..
Yahatahigashi–ku,
Kitakyus,
Fukuoka 805–002
Japan
Tel 09 36622080
Fax 0936622088
info@tilia.ne.jp

Lavander Aromatherapy Ltd
PO Box Lavender Aromatherapy LTD
23542
1683 Nicossia
Cyprus
Tel 0035722666870
Fax 0035722667104
lavanda@cytanet.com.cy

Natural Planter Co., Ltd
6F–1, No 118
Ta Tun 20 st
Taichung City
Taiwan
Tel 886 42 398984
Fax 886 42 329010
Ufjt0340@ms9.hinet.net

Sozo
8 Bencran Road
Beragh
Sixmilecross
Omagh
Tyrone
BT79 0SF
Sozo_serve@hotmail.com

Elaine Cooper
Walsall Hospice
Stoney Lane
Little Bloxwich
Walsall
West Midlands
WS3 3DW
Elaine.Cooper@walsall.nhs.uk

**London School of
   Complementary Health,**
3 Ivory Square,
Plantation Wharf,
London
SW11 3UE
gideonroberts@hotmail.com

Accrediting Bodies

Institute of Aromatic Medicine
Spa Villa
41 Leicester Road
Hinckley
Leicestershire
LE10 1LW
aromed@hotmail.com

**International Federation of
   Professional Aromatherapists**
82 Ashby Road
Hinckley
Leics
Tel: 01455 637987
Email: info@ifparoma.org

Index